Victory over Autism

Victory over Autism

Practical Steps and Wisdom toward
Recovery for the Whole Family

Mary Romaniec

Foreword by
Anju Iona Usman, MD, FAAFP,
ABIHM, Hom-C

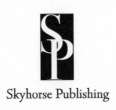

Skyhorse Publishing

Skyhorse Publishing books may be purchased in bulk at special discounts for sales promotion, corporate gifts, fund-raising, or educational purposes. Special editions can also be created to specifications. For details, contact the Special Sales Department, Skyhorse Publishing, 307 West 36th Street, 11th Floor, New York, NY 10018 or info@skyhorsepublishing.com.

Skyhorse® and Skyhorse Publishing® are registered trademarks of Skyhorse Publishing, Inc.®, a Delaware corporation.

Visit our website at www.skyhorsepublishing.com.

10 9 8 7 6 5 4 3 2 1

Library of Congress Cataloging-in-Publication Data is available on file.

Cover design by Brian Peterson
Cover photos: Thinkstock

Print ISBN: 978-1-63450-515-4
Ebook ISBN: 978-1-63450-845-2

Printed in the United States of America

Dedicated to the memory of
my nephew

Joshua Sway Derrick-Jones
December 5, 2010 – January 21, 2012

Contents

Foreword

When you hear that your child has been diagnosed with Autism, your whole life makes a serious adjustment. As you find yourself being forced to multitask at a new level it is natural to become hyper-focused, as your main priority now becomes to help your child heal. While this drive and dedication can be a great virtue in the battle against autism, it can also leach attention needed to nurture and address other aspects of your life. When you become so concentrated on researching doctors, finding therapists, and studying treatments, there is a tendency to unconsciously neglect the side effects that autism can have on your family. Having a child with autism can emotionally, socially, and financially impact your family, marriage, other children, and even your own well-being.

As a family physician, I have been caring for patients diagnosed with autism—as well as their families—for over fifteen years. I have had a front-row seat as the world has watched this epidemic unfold before our eyes. Being on the front lines of an epidemic that now affects 1 in 34 boys and 1 in 143 girls, I have struggled to help guide my patients and their families. I have incessantly read literature, conducted research, and attended think tanks. I have traveled around the world to discuss with parents, doctors, researchers, educators, and politicians about how to spread and exchange knowledge about this multifaceted disorder. I have incorporated diet, nutrition, nutraceuticals, herbs, essential oils, homeopathy, energy techniques, hyperbaric oxygen therapy, and detoxification strategies into my practice to hit every medical dimension of treating autism. However, in my search for medical answers, I have neglected one of the most important aspects of dealing with a chronic disorder such as autism: I have failed to attend to the mental, emotional, social, financial, physical, and spiritual impact it can have on each family. Only in the past few years have I realized the importance of tending to these secondary effects.

As a parent, I have been in your shoes. I have searched high and low for answers to help my own children. Although I do not have a child on the autism spectrum, I have three children with chronic medical and immune issues. Like you, I have exhausted all of my resources, time, and energy to help my children. Even with all my medical knowledge and hard work, I have struggled to address all aspects of each child's condition. My eldest daughter passed away from a peanut allergy, and my youngest daughter is living homebound as a result of dealing with multiple severe chemical sensitivities. By depleting my energy in dealing with sick children, financial obligations, and chronic stress, my marriage of twenty-six years has become a casualty. At times, I have felt hopeless, especially when my precious daughter passed away.

I know that when you are fighting for your child, it is easy to lose focus on your family, your other children, your marriage, and your own emotional needs. Yet, you will be surprised to learn that nurturing your other relationships and taking care of yourself is conducive to harmony in the home environment, and will actually help your sick child as an effect. Very few books have been written to confront these facets of autism. The question parents are faced with today is, "How can I help my child with autism while also helping my spouse, our other children, and—most importantly—myself?" In *Victory over Autism*, Mary Romaniec helps you navigate through your journey to help your child and family overcome the effects of autism. Whether you have just started your journey, or are further down the road, feeling defeated and desperate, know that you can find hope with the right tools. Hope is often considered a feeling. In my experience, however, it has been an active process.

In hindsight, I wish the tools and insights Mary provides in *Victory over Autism* had been provided to me when I was dealing with my personal and professional struggles. At this point in my life, I still work to care for sick patients, their families that have been torn apart, and my own children's illnesses. Throughout my journey, I have found that people and resources like Mary's book truly help guide and pull me through the tough times. There are days when the battle takes its toll, when I feel utterly defeated, but I know that, in the long run, there is a way to live this life and feel victorious in the end.

Anju Iona Usman, MD, FAAFP, ABIHM, Hom-C

Introduction

Not long ago, I sat at a lakeside beach as families splashed and played during a warm afternoon. In the midst of the happy sounds was the high-pierced cry of a child that I intuitively knew was on the autism spectrum, just from the decibel of his cry. I searched around for the child and his family at this beach, and sure enough, it was a toddler-aged boy that caught my attention earlier in the day because of how often he bolted from his mother. It's second nature in the veteran autism parent to recognize the symptoms when we see them. It was also second nature to go speak with the mother about her son and to offer some measure of information and hope in the course of the conversation.

That's my life—my mission, if you will; one parent at a time, multiplied by years of countless emails, phone calls, and private conversations. By the age of four, my son no longer met the diagnostic criteria for autism and was declared recovered by his pediatrician. Recovery does not mean the same thing as cured, however, because the underlying immunological issues will continue to exist and perhaps remain a lasting scar. But by all measures, Daniel is a typical teen, complete with the complexity of this age. He is also a testament to the endless possibilities ahead for the children being diagnosed today with autism.

There are many others who count themselves blessed with recovery for their child too. There are also many more families who can't claim recovery yet but still give of their time to speak to another parent who has just received the news that their child has autism. The science of understanding the nature and comorbidities of autism is just beginning to grow, as are the available treatment options. More importantly has been the growth in parental awareness that autism is treatable.

Critics of this book will undoubtedly be in the camp that autism is not a "disease" or "disorder" but rather just a difference to be embraced. That is where we part ways. Autism is medical, and parents around the world have had to come to this realization, often without the help of traditional medicine. It is not just genetics playing a role in the levels of autism we see today. Many of us believe that environment, foods, and a bloated vaccine schedule have sent the genetically predisposed over the cliff into immune system dysfunction . . . with a cascade of side effects that lands them somewhere on the autism spectrum and all of the other comorbidities associated with chronic ill health.

No matter where you stand on the topic of what causes autism, the focus of this book is to get you, the parent or caregiver, on the path to finding the answers to better health for your child. The purpose of this book then is to instill confidence on the path ahead, and provide an understanding of who you become in the process and what you will undoubtedly endure as an individual, a couple, and a family in the journey of overcoming autism. What you will mainly overcome is the impact autism has on your family.

Writing this book was not easy. For every word written, there was a reminder of how much more needed to be said to parents who were just discovering that their child had autism. This book was born from the conviction that too few families are given straight answers and even fewer are given any measure of hope that their child will improve or recover fully, as my son did.

My gratitude for this journey for our son's return to health is boundless. Our family and friends have born witness to the miracle of the possible, wrapped in hope in a boy who proved that autism is treatable and that children can recover. Just before he turned eleven years old, Daniel was invited to be a speaker at the benefit banquet at Autism One in Chicago to give a small presentation on his recovery. Long before the days of internet saturation, I made the decision to write his story of recovering from autism for a magazine. Daniel's name has been out there for a long time now, so the genie cannot be put back in the bottle.

It did not occur to me then that there may be a time I would regret not using a pseudonym for him. After all, he would one day be a job seeker, and the stigma of once having autism might follow him (sad there is any stigma at all). But Daniel turned to me and said, "Mom, this is why I came. This is my mission, so that you can go do your mission. Now go finish your book." There are times when our children leave us speechless, and this was one such time. That night, I had the privilege of introducing him at the podium to a crowd of over three hundred and fifty adults, mostly parents of children with autism.

I was reminded of how far he had come, a boy who at one time was destined for an institution, if the doctors' predictions proved accurate. I remembered the sleepless nights, the therapies, procedures, and everything else in between that he gratefully forgot. But that night I remembered how he always made me proud to be his mother. Speaking with a cadence of a mature young boy as he scrolled through the PowerPoint, he made me and others cry for what he was doing so innocently at that podium. He was instilling hope in all of us, and giving the parents there the wherewithal to "go do their mission" too.

Our story of recovery is real. The fact that improvement or recovery from autism is not widely known in the medical community or general public is baffling. Even though countless children have recovered or improved significantly, skepticism still reigns. Why this is can only be explained by how autism remains a disorder that is not understood, both in medical establishments as well as the general public, with the word "recovered" relegated to defining a hopeful desire, not a reality in autism.

Still, a legion of parents has declared war on autism, refusing to accept the grim prognosis and scant medical information. And they are making a difference in their children's well-being, astounding medical and educational experts with their child's improved health and progress.

Information about treatment options is not common in medical protocols or procedures that your traditional doctor embraces. There are pockets of doctors who have availed themselves of the latest research, but they often rely on excerpts to bring their entire understanding on a medical condition up to speed. You are in good company if you are even thinking about pursuing recovery for your child—or at least a child who is free from pain and is functioning better cognitively. All of this is yours for the asking—simply by understanding how you have the ability to be that difference in your child's life.

Fear of the unknown mixed with daunting decisions that must be made after a child is diagnosed, can be insidious if we let it. This is why many parents don't take the first step to finding better health answers for their child. It takes courage. It takes trust in your own abilities to find what your child needs to improve their social, emotional, cognitive, behavioral, and physical well-being.

If you are a physician or therapist reading this book for the benefit of your patients, then thank you for caring enough to want to help, or even just understand. The most important thing you can and should offer is encouragement, so that the parents can work towards helping their children heal, either with your help or the help of others. Yes, there are limits to the things physicians can support, but simply listening with a genuine sense of caring will go a long way to helping parents cope through the unbridled challenges from their child and resulting family dynamics.

As savvy resourceful parents, we have come to believe a core mantra about ourselves: *we are the link* to our child's future. These same parents have become each other's mentors to provide the information they desperately need to help their children. They also have become mentors to physicians and educators, determined to bring autism treatment awareness into the mainstream. Now it is time to bring this same message to other parents who need to know they too have the ability, and the responsibility, to be the difference in their child's life.

Indeed, *WE are the missing link.*

While I tell the stories of other parents and children, I have been mindful of how they want to be known, whether by their real names, first name only, or pseudonym (denoted with a *). I am deeply grateful they allowed me to tell their stories, and I will honor their need for privacy.

Chapter One

The Childhood Imagined Has Changed: The Grief Cycle and Autism Explained

Let's face it, when we were planning our lives after college graduation none of us planned on autism to be a part of our future. Ideally, we graduated, got a job, maybe traveled and experienced life, and then fell in love enough to marry. Our dream life unfolded with a child on the way, and more later. All was well in our little world . . . until it actually wasn't.

Our child is diagnosed with autism and our entire perspective of what life was supposed to be like becomes a mirage. Our children were supposed to have friends, sleepovers, attend birthday parties, have dance recitals, get a driver's license, go to prom and then to college. They were supposed to go on to have successful lives and children of their own. But the milestones that we thought we would celebrate change in an instant.

We listen to soccer sideline conversations and we wonder how our lives segued so far off the course of what we imagined for our children, the ones struggling to keep up with the other children on the field. We wonder if we were ever as shallow in our priorities as our friends and neighbors now appear to us, or whether we are now a different breed of parent. In this dichotomy, we come to grieve. This chapter then explains why and how the grief cycle impacts most of us emotionally, psychologically, and physically, and why these stages are necessary to transform us into bold individuals who make a difference rather than sink into unresolved despair.

Grief happens to all of us at some point in our lives. Whether we grieve the death of a loved one, the loss of a marriage, or even the loss of social status, we all grieve to varying degrees. With the autism diagnosis and each missed milestone, we grieve the loss of the childhood we imagined for our child. We also grieve our own sense of failure that tightens around us to create a sense of helplessness. In a small way, we grieve who we used to be, at a time when our world was not filled with relentless stress and anxiety. We also grieve the unknown, the future that is no longer defined for our child or for us.

I have spent countless hours in the throes of the grief cycle; first my own, and then my husband's, followed by the numerous parents I mentored over the years as they navigated through their own grief. There is a pattern to our grief as autism parents, one that has not been defined by conventional psychology. Since I am a huge fan of Dr. Elisabeth Kubler-Ross, who eloquently explained the cycles of grief in her book *On Death and Dying,* I parlayed her findings into the kind of grief parents go through when their child is diagnosed with autism.

Instead of the stages associated with death—denial, anger, bargaining, depression, acceptance—autism has its own unique grief cycle. After a child receives the diagnosis, the parents begin the process of coming to grips with the prognosis of their child, which encompasses the loss of the childhood that the parent imagined for their child. *Fear* is followed by *denial, anger, bargaining/guilt* interchangeably, *acceptance,* and finally *resolve* to overcome the impact of autism on the family. The problems with mental and emotional health happen when a parent or caregiver gets stuck in the first four stages and does not progress to the final two stages, lost in the mire of grief-related inertia.

The Path of Despair Has Exit Signs along the Way

When Daniel was diagnosed, we received the ominous prognosis of no hope, no cure, and a group home in his future. But the diagnosis was not the problem as much as the day-to-day behaviors and health issues we were dealing with. When your child is banging his head on the floor, smearing feces on the walls, and writhing in agony, you intuitively head in the direction of fixing your child's pain, only to be met by an uninterested or unknowing physician that attributes any and all symptoms to your child's autism, as though they cease to exist with the label as a moniker—"autistic child."

But the path of despair does indeed have exit signs along the way. Rather than making this sound like artful "feel good" words, I will point out the obvious—kids are recovering from autism! And your child can be one of them. You will probably go through hell to make this happen. Chances are you already are going through hell. The difference is that your child and family have the possibility of declaring victory over autism and celebrating the milestones you always imagined.

Grief stages are not widely discussed in the autism community. If they were, I am convinced there would be less of a sense of isolation that leads to desperate acts. This is not to say that mental health issues would not happen. The grief cycle is ever present and universal to all who have a child with the diagnosis of autism, albeit in varying degrees. What is crucial is how we choose to work through it in order to get to the stage of *resolve*. If we don't, we end up on a slippery slope toward relentless hopelessness. And that leads to greater consequences, which we see unfolding in the autism community at alarming rates.

When Grief Is Unresolved—A New Crisis!

Imagine being a poor, single mother whose dream life has been dashed many times over, and then her child is diagnosed with autism. In her despair, the young mother feels the weight of the difficult life ahead for her son, and she is driven to the breaking point. In July, 2010, a single mother from the Bronx did the unthinkable: she killed her twelve-year-old son who had autism, and then killed herself. A note left behind explained her untenable situation of trying to care for her son while trying to overcome her own sense of growing desolation. She hoped Jesus would forgive her sins. With this act she became another statistic of "parent who kills their child afflicted with autism," often killing themselves too. It is not an anomaly. It is a sad trend.

A few months earlier, a married father from Maine shot his adult son with autism and then turned the gun on himself, leaving a suicide note stating he could not stand the idea of what would happen to his son once his parents were no longer there to care for him.

When I lived in California, there was a local single mother with a middle school–aged son who had an overt need to wear his beanie every day. It was his comfort. Even though it was against middle school rules, the mother pleaded with the district to allow her son to wear the hat. But the district refused. For this mother, it was the final straw of feeling the rejection levied against her son, and that night she took a gun to him and then to herself. Surprisingly, they both lived, but she was brought up on attempted murder charges and her son was placed in state custody.

Stories of murder/suicide involving a child with autism being killed by a parent abound all over the country, if not the world. What is not explained to those who do not have a child with autism is the overwhelming grief that accompanies the diagnosis of autism, and the ensuing years of coping with the child's health and behavior issues. It is a cycle of almost blind despair as parents go through the grief process, followed by hope—if the cycle is allowed to complete itself. In this case, the hopeful answers for these parents were not there, and unmitigated grief consumed them. The autism community is left to find the answers and ask the broader questions of why this continues to happen, and what to do about it.

The plight of Alex Spourdalakis galvanized the autism community in 2013 when his story of hospital abuse made international headlines. Admitted to the hospital in February 2013, his mother Dorothy was desperate to find answers to what was causing his gastrointestinal pain, and to relieve her non-verbal fourteen-year-old son's obvious misery. Instead of receiving treatments, he was restrained to a hospital bed and covered with only a bed sheet while he continued to writhe in pain. He was not even afforded the most basic standards of medical testing or care, with the excuse that "autism is a mystery" being used by hospital staff as a reason to ignore his obvious distress. His mother's pleas for help to address her son's significant gastrointestinal distress were ignored.

As a mother, I was gripped by her situation, appalled by the hospital staff's ignorance about the physical components of autism, one of them being gastrointestinal issues. How could they not know that Alex was in pain? How could they not offer basic medical services to this boy or offer comforting words of reassurance to the mother? In the autism community, there was a sense of disbelief that this sad trend in traditional medicine was continuing. We all had stories of one kind or another on ignorance from the medical community, but this situation was over the top, and we became galvanized as a community. We wrote letters, made phone calls, and rallied to get this boy dismissed from the hospital in order to get him real treatment from doctors who understood that autism is medical, not psychological with just a nuanced difference in behaviors.

Alex was eventually released and privately sponsored to be seen by a well-known gastroenterologist who specialized in treating children with autism. Reports and a video that surfaced later proved what the rest of us intuitively knew was happening to Alex: his gut was a mess, full of ulcers and inflammation. Dorothy was shown in the video with tears, shaking her head. Despite validation from the doctor with a new way of treating Alex, her despair and desperation remained.

In spite of the confirmation that the severe gastrointestinal issues were contributing to Alex's pain, Dorothy's sense of her situation after years of seeking answers were still untenable; as was her mental stability. On June 9, 2013, Dorothy and her friend Agatha Skrodzka killed Alex; drugging him, slitting his wrists, and then stabbing him in the heart. They then tried to kill themselves by overdosing on sleeping pills, but they survived and were charged with first degree murder.

Facebook posts by activists close to Dorothy spoke of their growing concern for her and Alex. But nothing could have prepared them for this final act of desperation. Many in the autism community were dumbfounded. She was finally getting him some help, or so we thought. What would prompt a parent to do this to their own child? Ultimately, we asked who was responsible. Was it Dorothy? The ignorant medical community? The hospital? Or was it the autism community for not doing enough to get information or resources into the hands of parents like Dorothy sooner?

The Six Stages of Grief

Fear

I had been acquainted with Laura for twenty years and knew her as a vivacious woman with creative talents, which is why the tremble in her voice was disturbing. She had the sound of a woman who was to face the executioner: desperate, but with a constraint in her voice that told me she needed to be stoic, if only for her own dignity. And I would never forget how she changed my life with one phone call.

She had just returned from a well-known pediatric hospital where the leading neurologist had just diagnosed Laura's son with pervasive developmental disorder, not otherwise specified (PDD-NOS), coupled with a horrific prognosis for his future. Even though it is understood that PDD-NOS carries with it the inference that it is a "milder" form of autism, this physician declared that her son would one day be institutionalized, would never be professionally productive, and that Laura and her husband should get ready for the pending divorce because it went hand in hand with the autism diagnosis.

Now I understood why her trembling voice was nothing more than disguised terror. At that moment, she needed someone to save her and her family from certain "death." After I spoke with her and gave her valid information that would make a difference in the well-being of her son, the tremor in her voice was replaced with a bit of lightness. It must have made a difference because the next day she called me with another friend on the phone who had just had the same experience with her son's doctor. She asked me to repeat what I had said to her the day before, only this time it was Laura who was pushing past her fear to uplift her friend.

This is our reality. Our child receives a diagnosis from the physician and we are left to grapple with the consequences of having no information or the wrong information, as a natural response to what physicians do not know about autism. This includes the parent who is a physician too. I am one of many autism parent mentors who have had to educate physicians on *their* child. We provide them the same information and tenets of hope that belies their profession. We can, as parents, because we are not stymied by protocol, nor do we dispense medical advice beyond our own experiences with our children or what we have learned by attending conferences and seminars. *Fear*, then, is the first stage in the grief cycle, and it can paralyze a parent permanently, or propel them forward as it did me.

One of the families I mentored had two physician parents; the mother a neurologist and the father an anesthesiologist. I sat next to the father at a conference and struck up a conversation, explaining that my son was undergoing intravenous immuno-globulin (IVIG) treatments as well as other therapies and was making tremendous progress. He asked me to speak with his wife so she could hear our story of success. Mainly, he wanted her to be supportive of moving forward with treatments, which was why they were both at this autism conference. She was hesitant, he explained, because her medical training called for double-blind placebo studies followed by clinical trials followed by more studies before submitting to her son receiving any treatments. Her husband relayed that it was causing friction in the marriage because he believed she was using her medical training as an excuse to not make any decisions, out of fear of making the wrong decision. She was a neurologist who admitted that she had not studied autism in medical school, which is why her traditional medicine training was failing her now.

I understood her trepidation, but I also understood the father's sense of urgency to begin some kind of treatment. When I met his wife she was gracious and full of purpose to learn all she could about autism treatments, including our experience with IVIG. As I told her how the local immunologist had carefully screened our son for this particular treatment, I also spoke about the experiences we had as parents as we helped our son overcome some of the treatment's side effects I added in other considerations of what to expect while a child receives IVIG, the same ones I have listed for every parent who has asked. There was nothing overly medical about this conversation other than our experiences and a recommendation to schedule an appointment to speak with the immunologist, which she agreed to do.

I ran into this couple about six months later and found out that their son had indeed been a good candidate for the treatment, so they began IVIG and saw a positive response in his health. But in spite of the great progress from the treatment, the mother once again fell on her medical training background and stopped all further treatments until there were more studies done, much to the angst of the father, who seemed resolved to move forward. The mother meant well for her son, but she became paralyzed by the fear of the unknown and was therefore unable to make any kind of decision. I have seen this in every parent in varying forms. Fear can paralyze decision making, over and over again.

In my case, I feared the consequences of *not* doing something—anything—to stop my son's pain. Receiving the diagnosis was nothing in comparison to the child who woke at two in the morning screaming in pain; or the child who banged his head, arched his back in agony, and flat out wailed for ninety minutes after every nap. No, I feared his cries of pain more than I feared the treatments to end the pain. So, I was propelled by that kind of fear, so much so that I almost skipped the next stage in the grief cycle: denial.

Denial

In the autism community there is an odd phenomenon of parents in denial that their child even has autism, choosing to not seek a diagnosis for *fear* that their child will be stigmatized with a label. In other words, the diagnosis will make it more real and something they will then need to acknowledge, deal with, announce to their relatives, etc. They make excuses for their child's behavior, become angry or distant, or in some way ignore the implications of their child's ill health and autism-related behaviors. There was a time when parents in our community would hesitate to say something to another parent on their suspicions of autism, especially to total strangers. But the number of autism cases is escalating, autism awareness is more acceptable, and parents of affected children are becoming bolder in their approach to the next parent whose child they suspect has autism. Actually, we are outright audacious at times.

Denial takes other forms, as it did with my husband Richard. For him, just saying the word "autism" was difficult and he could not put it in the same sentence with his son's name for over a year after the diagnosis. When we sought a second opinion at a well-known pediatric facility, the neurologist there declared that, while he didn't know a whole lot about autism, he did know that some of these kids "just snap out of it." Rich thought this doctor was golden since he had determined that our son would, in essence, just come to his senses one day. I knew the doctor was an idiot, and said so. Clearly, we did not share the same perspective.

Denial was also apparent in the way a parent would tell me that their child was "higher functioning" or only "mild," so no treatments or therapies would be necessary. But the health issues remained and escalated as the child got older, so that a once high-functioning child often eventually became a teenager with significant mental health issues. The tough cases were when I would receive a phone call from a parent who would relay that the other parent was in denial and becoming belligerent in their insistence that a child did not have autism. Or they acknowledged the autism but determined that no medical treatments or therapy would work so they would not support any effort along these lines. Those were the families that would see the roughest waters when this grief stage of denial would cascade around the marriage and affect the entire family.

In one instance, I received a call from a desperate grandmother whose daughter and son-in-law refused any and all treatments for their child with autism because it "cost too much" to treat him. She then cried that they had no problems putting in a pool but her own grandson was ignored medically. That wasn't denial as much as flat out neglect, and it broke my heart. There is a story that circulates occasionally in the autism community of a certain celebrity that decided to focus on their movie career instead of helping their child with autism. The boy was put into a group home at a young age and the celebrity went on to an illustrious career. Little was ever mentioned in the press about this boy. Denial takes many forms.

One mother told me she was taking her son to a local children's hospital to have him possibly diagnosed with autism.

While I welcomed her proactive approach, I knew the effort was going to end at just getting the diagnosis. The implications of the diagnosis were given the same level of importance as a mild case of the flu, meaning her form of denial was to take a very casual attitude and continue on with their lives as if it didn't matter. I knew it would matter one day.

One of the worst kinds of denial to deal with is the ones from the physicians and school psychologists who are usually the first ones who must suggest either a diagnosis or an evaluation for a diagnosis. But when the local experts refuse to acknowledge a child is in need of a diagnosis or evaluations, it becomes tremendously difficult to obtain the necessary services. Too often we hear from parents who would continuously tell the pediatrician or other doctor that something was wrong with their child, only to have the concern dismissed with, "That's because he's a boy" or "It's just a phase she is going through."

In Daniel's case, I was at the pediatrician's office every other week begging the doctor for answers to why Daniel was crying continuously and had non-stop diarrhea. It was not until a few months later that his physical therapist suggested that Daniel be evaluated for autism spectrum disorder. This was when his symptoms of sensory issues, odd behaviors and developmental delays began to be explained. We delivered the news later to the well-meaning pediatrician, who was at a loss as to what to suggest to us going forward. He told us he had not studied more than a paragraph on autism in medical school, and his wife was still looking for answers for his two children on the spectrum.

When a school district denies having a child evaluated they will say something like, "But your child is making adequate progress" as a way of signaling they don't want to evaluate a child or provide services. Even when parents bring in outside evaluations with the full diagnosis, some school districts will choose to ignore the medical recommendations and either refuse further evaluations or a follow up IEP meeting (all of which is completely illegal). This is one of the reasons why parents feel marginalized by the school districts and remain on guard. This is not every school district but a swath of them. And their denial is what leads to a child getting further behind, leading a parent further down the next path of the grief cycle: anger. With school district interactions, the anger phase can come up over and over.

Anger

It is only fair to bring up the *anger* stage by showcasing how my own anger spilled in every direction, only I didn't exactly know it at the time. I was superwoman on steroids cleaning the house to get ready for the therapists of the day, or the mom taking her kids to the playground in between doctors' appointments or some other chore that had autism spelled all over it. Even my rushed movements to clean the house carried an element of anger, which eventually led to a breakdown in my health.

Rich would come home, and for some reason I would choose the moment he walked in the door to just spill out the day's events, so he got the brunt end of it. Staying up late, getting up early, and eating crappy food did little to balance out my mood, so it was not hard for Rich to tick me off, which then led to further stress and anxiety that erupted into fights. Rich was navigating his own anger cycle, too, so the two of us were easily pushing each other's buttons. Gratefully, I knew several like-minded autism moms who were all going through the anger stage simultaneously, which allowed us to vent with another parent who understood the upheaval that was affecting our lives.

Parents of children with autism are also angry at the medical establishment who we believe either harmed our children, treated them badly, offered us no information, and in all other ways let us down. That kind of anger is tough to get over, as is the anger toward school districts that we deem to be more concerned with their bottom line than the kids they are supposed to serve. This is why the anger stage is a tough one to push through: it keeps rearing its head and we are like the knights heading into battle against the bureaucratic dragon all over again.

There are a lot of tremendous activist parents in the autism community. There are also a lot of parents who are using their anger to propel them to a greater mission of ensuring the next generation of parents understands all of the things they wish they had known before their child developed autism (yes, I use the word developed as opposed to "born with" autism). For them, anger over the outrage of loss is strength, giving structure and purpose to their lives. But at times they get stuck in their anger and rally around the autism cause more so than getting their child the appropriate treatments. The anger stage must be pushed through so that it becomes manageable enough to ignore when you must turn your attention to what matters most—your child's well-being.

I was working with the father of two severely affected boys and he asked me to speak to their mother, his former wife. He was hopeful that they could come to some sort of truce, enough to start making decisions together on medical treatments for their sons. He videotaped doctors' appointments and would have her review them after, carefully choosing his words so as not to disparage her in any way. Unfortunately, the same could not be said for her. She used every opportunity during our phone call to belittle the father's efforts, to count her pain from the divorce, and to pick at her anger as fodder to use against her former husband. She was completely stuck in the anger stage. All of this cost her and the boys dearly. The boys in particular suffered as a result since the mother opted to block any and all treatments for them and threatened to drag the father back into court to seek full custody. This is not an uncommon occurrence.

There were also the phone calls I would receive from the mothers who would ask me to speak to their former spouse about the necessary diet changes (these were the really tough calls to handle). Apparently, just the idea that the information was coming from someone other than the former spouse made the message more believable. Truthfully, I saw this with a lot of married couples too, where diet changes and therapies were resisted until someone other than the spouse talked about it. One of these spouses was a doctor who asked me to speak to his wife about the diet changes that were needed. His own colleagues couldn't be counted on to understand nutrition he explained, and they would criticize his effort to help his son. So he thought another mother would be able to convey the information better than he could since they were both just muddling through the diagnosis. He too expressed tremendous disappointment and anger toward his own profession for their attitude and the lack of information on treatments and therapies. But he pushed forward through the anger stage by reaching out to find the answers where he could.

Then there was the middle-of-the-night phone call from an anxious mother who had started dietary intervention, but when her husband objected the child was put back on the old diet of heavily processed foods, which caused significant gastrointestinal pain. She called urgently to ask what remedy to give her son to alleviate the pain, all while her husband was yelling at her to put the phone down and help him with their distraught child. At this point I could not help her since she was navigating her own grief while managing the behaviors of both her husband and her son. This was one of those parents I knew would remain in the grief cycle for longer than usual, and hopefully one day move to a stage where the real changes begin to happen.

Bargaining/Guilt

In the original description of the grief cycle described by Dr. Kubler-Ross, she lists bargaining and depression as two separate stages in the grief cycle. In autism, we combine bargaining and guilt because of how we use the two simultaneously, and then separately, taking turns on the pendulum between forward action and guilt-filled emotions.

In the grief cycle, *bargaining* presents itself as doing a little bit of effort thinking that at least you are doing something so maybe you really don't have to commit fully to a holistic effort, whether it is doing research, starting a new diet or treatment protocol, or just writing a simple letter to the school district. We soon realize that our mediocre effort is not enough, and this leads to guilt in varying degrees, potentially leading to guilt becoming our narcotic of choice that gets us up in the morning. This was me, a flat out "guiltaholic." I was also an incessant bargainer in my quest to find the answers for my son, without really wanting to do the hard work once I found them.

Thankfully, I lingered in *bargaining* for less than a year before I finally understood what I had to do. *Guilt*, on the other hand, followed me as a reminder of all I had "done wrong" to hurt my son, and every day was a reminder that I had the duty to make it up to him in some way. Sounds crazy doesn't it? But I know I am not alone in this perverse thinking. It's endemic in our community that mothers in particular gravitate to the drug of guilt. I have yet to meet a mother on this journey who did not languish with guilt as a bedfellow for a while, or still does. I wondered about what I had done to my body before pregnancy to possibly cause harm to my unborn child; coupled with the pregnancy and labor complications that may have added to his health issues. A myriad of thoughts ran through my head on everything I would have done differently to spare my son unnecessary pain. And at other times I am in thunderstruck on how Daniel's autism changed me for the better and propelled me on the mission to help other families. Still, I would have given anything to not have him suffer.

If I had a bargain to make with God, it was this: "Dear God, help me to find the answers for my son. Point me in the right direction and I will follow. If there is a door, I will knock it in. If it is a window, I will crash through it. Just know that I will do whatever it takes to help my son. I just need you to show me the way."

Many of us bargain with God after we have been angry first. When Daniel was first diagnosed, I was contacted by a family friend who said he was petitioning to use Daniel as a possible "miracle case" for someone he thought should be canonized by the Catholic Church. In the Catholic Church, it means that someone who has been deemed holy enough to possibly make it into Heaven must now have three clear miracles attributed to their intercession in order to be canonized and made a saint.

Even as a lifelong Catholic, I was incensed. While I did not mind prayers for my son I was not going to proclaim his progress to be the direct result of some divine miracle. I welcome miracles in all forms except the ones that stipulate that only God can cure, or offer recovery. This is not meant as an affront to those of faith, but a reality check on how miracles happen—you go make them happen! I would often say, "I prayed as if everything depended on God and worked as if everything depended on me. And, together, God and I made a pretty good team." Okay, the phrase was probably borrowed from some other saint but the point was that the miracle was ours for the doing, not just the asking.

When I mentored other parents who leaned in the direction of wanting to just pray for a miracle I would caution them firmly and tell them to choose the miracle and go make it happen. And they did.

My *bargaining* stage stopped after I committed fully to diet changes for my son without deviating, for a full three weeks. We saw tremendous gains, so much so that I thought, "Whew, out of the woods, going back to feeding him some of his old diet now." BIG mistake. Within three weeks, the cause and effect of a little gluten food here a little there meant that he was now in full regression—and it was worse than before. He once again woke up screaming in pain, repetitively banged his head on the wall, and planted his face into the floor. He had just turned two, so this time frame is stuck in my head as the peak of the worst days we experienced with autism.

Looking back now, I still can't believe I took him to occupational therapy in this condition, and on this particular day. I reasoned that it was just a bad day and he would be fine once he was in therapy. Was I ever wrong. The entire session was a waste. The occupational therapist asked me what happened and wondered if it was a new drug setting him off because he had lost six months of progress literally overnight.

I answered that yes, it was a new drug and the drug was food, and I was a bona fide terrible mother for feeding it to him. I meant every word, calling Rich to repeat the morning's events and my conversation with the therapist. I then screamed into the phone, "I am a horrible mother! I did this to him!" Nothing Rich could say was going to convince me otherwise so he just asked, "What can I do to help?"

I told him that I was going to the local health food store to get stocked up on any and all gluten/dairy-free food items so that Daniel never suffered like this again—and I was going to spend A LOT of money, I told Rich. Money was a big issue with us, so this was almost a dare because, in this instance, money was going to take the back seat to what Daniel needed. Rich always agreed with me when it came to what the kids needed, so he offered his full support. Frankly, I think he was worried about my mental state after the phone call. He rarely heard me cry, let alone tell him that I was a crappy mother.

So my *bargaining* stopped, but only because my *guilt* overwhelmed and motivated me forward. I will elaborate more on the toxic soup we create with guilt in chapter 7 since we all know it deserves so much more than a paragraph of explanation. There is also a portion on what to do as guiltaholics to manage our addiction to this emotion. After this breakdown and cathartic understanding of my role in getting Daniel better, I was led to the next stage in the grief cycle: *acceptance*.

Acceptance

Acceptance is the interesting stage. It brings with it the perception that "all is well in the world" because someone has accepted their lot in life for what it is and finds little can be done to change anything to make it better or even different. They are in *acceptance* because the grief cycle has brought them to this point, and maybe that is truly where they will remain due to circumstances in their life. Or perhaps the serious health issues of their child keep them from moving beyond this stage. There are plenty of autism families who have processed through all of the grief stages, made heroic efforts to advocate fully on behalf of their child, and circle back to this stage because this is where the cycle has finally landed, as it should.

The version of *acceptance* that I cannot support is the one that embraces the perspective that there is no hope and no cure, so it's not worth trying to do anything. Parents who adhere to this line of thought believe that the child with autism should simply be accepted for who they are (ignoring all the comorbid health issues, of course). They believe that autism should be celebrated. Um, no thank you. I will celebrate children, but never autism, for what autism did to my son and our family and the families of countless others. While some families look at autism as a "gift," I look at the children as the gift, not the autism. Many of us in the autism community find it absurd that autism has the word celebrate next to it as a measure toward acceptance. Can you imagine if the word autism was replaced with cancer, diabetes, asthma, peanut allergies, or some other serious disorder or illness? There would be outrage at the whole idea that something that causes so much pain would be "celebrated."

There is a huge divide in our community on this whole concept of what is considered *acceptance*. I have had online back and forth responses with other parents who wear the badge of acceptance with pride, but also brandish it as a mantra that the rest of us should follow since to them it is a greater form of love to just accept our children for who they are. I am sure they meant well, but for those of us who have declared war on what robbed us of the lives we imagined for our children it is an affront to ask us to do the same, especially when our children are suffering.

My first venture to an autism support group was all about accepting that we as parents were helpless to help our children, but the parents with older affected children would hold our hands and tell us that they were there for us. They provided no information and looked at me cross-eyed when I asked about diet or school district help. That wasn't their purpose, they said. As one new mother wondered if she had bad karma and that was why she was "cursed" with a child with autism, the others only nodded their heads in sympathy. I was turned off and disgusted at this approach and knew that, no matter what, this would not be the form of support I would ever seek, or offer another parent. No, I needed information. Fast.

My own path to defining *acceptance* involved acknowledging that my role in my son's health and well-being had to change, and I had to take the lead. This was when my research efforts took on a whole new energy, a chaotic energy mixed with a whole bunch of determination to find the answers to help relieve Daniel's pain and developmental delays. With the Law of Attraction principles of just asking for the answers at my back, it seemed that *acceptance* was just a stepping stone to the final stage of the grief cycle: *resolve*.

This was when I met the parents who changed everything I ever thought about autism, and began to lead me to the whole idea that hope is real and that kids had the chance to get better. This was also when I met Lisa Ackerman of Talk About Curing Autism (TACA), which, at the time, was a highly informal group sitting in her living room in Huntington Beach,

California. The group consisted of other local parents who were trying to find answers for their children too. All we did was talk about what was working for our children and share resource information. But that was all it took. I was hooked. These were my people, my tribe, and together we were going to begin changing how autism was treated, one child at a time. To know that other parents were doing things that were helping, and that I could do the same, was the final energy drink I needed to move forward.

I finally *resolved* to overcome autism's grip on my son, step by step. Hanging out with TACA parents would be my vitamin of choice, mixed with my narcotic of daily guilt, to keep me going and find the answers for Daniel.

Resolve

Coming to this final stage was not all that climatic, as if I woke up one day and resolved to help my son overcome autism. It was more seamless, where one step of helping Daniel led to the next step until I suddenly began to see the prospect of our son fully recovering from autism.

It's this way with other families who have a child recovered too. It begins with a simple step like changing the child's diet or starting a new therapy. And when the positive changes show up in the child, the parent then wonders what else they can do to make a difference; daring to wonder if recovery might be for their child too. As more and more treatments and therapies become available, the idea that our kids can get better is picking up steam. Even if a child is not necessarily destined for full recovery, parents are grasping that their child can indeed improve and become healthier.

At an autism conference, I happened to meet a woman at breakfast with whom I struck up a conversation. She told me about her plans to look further into adult services since her son was now in his late teens and she needed to make arrangements for his long-term care. I don't know what prompted me to mention a new treatment protocol I had heard about to this new acquaintance, other than I knew she needed to attend the presentation about to be given on the topic. She hesitated a bit because she had a different mindset about the path she needed to take, and I understood that entirely. But in a flash, a wave of inspiration came over her and she grabbed her handbag and headed to the talk. Again, not knowing much about this protocol except what I had heard from others, I headed to the talk as well.

In this presentation there must have been several hundred parents, all eager to hear about this protocol that was showing so much promise but kicking up the controversy with it. As the presentation continued, there were slides of even the *older* children and adults who were improving. I looked over at my new friend and we both gleamed with that feeling of knowing she was meant to be in this presentation.

I ran into her later and she told me she had been in her room researching all day. Her entire perspective had changed. She was now *resolved* all over again. She still pursued information on the adult services, but this was being done in conjunction with something new, including a renewed sense of hope for a healthier child.

Recycling the Cycle

The thing about the grief cycle is that we almost certainly recycle through the cycle more than once. If your child has a setback, it is easy to get sucked right back into *fear*. Your child has a seizure, and there is almost a guarantee that the cycle will begin again: *fear, denial, anger, bargaining/guilt, acceptance, resolve to overcome*.

The point is that once you process through it the first time, the grief cycle seems to have a shorter time span between stages. All of this sounds fairly unscientific and generic except that I have seen this play out in the lives of families over and over. Think how often we are hit with a setback in our child's health, only to end up experiencing the same old emotions of fear, denial, anger, and bargaining/guilt to remind us what post-traumatic stress disorder feels like. Still, we carry on with our own tattered anxiety levels for the sake of our children. This is why the stress level of parents of special needs children is equated with combat stress. We are in a chronic stress situation.

It is how we understand and navigate through these stages that is important. It took me a while to understand that what was happening to me and Rich was grief-related. It took having grief impact our marriage to finally get a grip on the roller coaster of emotions. And I saw this same pattern play out in other individuals and couples, as well as the other siblings in the family. So when I began to mentor others on grief it became a sense of relief to them to know that the stages were temporary and with explanation.

This kind of cyclic grief is not just relegated to families who have a child with autism; it seems to correlate with any disorder that requires long-term care and treatment. The rest of this book will demonstrate how grief manifests itself, but it will also show how to overcome the impact it has on your life.

Tips for Understanding the Grief Cycle

Half of the battle with grief and autism is just to know these stages exist and that you are not alone in going through them. What you and your spouse are going through is completely normal, even if you don't think so at the time. Grief, as defined in this chapter, is necessary and serves a purpose for something better to come.

Here, then, is a recap on how to view the grief cycle you may be going through on the path to better days and better decision-making ahead for your child and family.

1. Grief is universal to us all, but in varying degrees. In autism, the parental grief cycle takes on additional stages of emotion beyond the grief associated with death.

2. Grief stages are for the most part temporary, but they appear more than once in cycle order, or in single stages, as the health issues of our child continue and the personal relationships of the family dynamic are affected. All of this is normal with grief and autism.

3. With autism comes a mountain of decisions that must be made, seemingly at the same time. It is the overwhelming nature of these decisions that can send a parent into the higher levels of stress, which leads to getting stuck in some part of the grief cycle.

4. Family dynamics are affected by the grief cycle, including the marriage and siblings of the affected child.

5. Grief has a physical component to it that leads to ill health of those going through it.

6. Overcoming grief's grip is what propels us forward as we begin to find the answers that benefit our child.

7. There is no set time on how long it takes to process through the grief cycles, but real progress does not begin until one or both of the parents reaches *resolve*.

8. The purpose of grief is to relinquish and mourn what we imagined for our child, and move us into a new reality of finding answers.

9. The fortitude we develop as we process through grief strengthens our resolve.

10. Grief changes who we are, leading us to overcome our personal, self-imposed obstacles, which eventually leads to greater understanding on what we must do as parents fighting for our children's future.

Chapter Two

The Necessary Attributes of the Bold Parent

The group of education professionals thought they had heard it all before, but the woman in front of them was different. Her voice was firm and her intent unquestionable. Her two-and-a-half year old son would *recover* from autism, and they would all be witnesses to the miracle unfolding before them. A sputtering cough from one said what they were thinking: clearly this mother was in denial because the label of autism predisposed this child to a lifetime of academic and lifestyle support. But they indulged this mother, if only for the seriousness of her expression.

That mother was me. And this is how the school district was put on notice that as a parent, I would be someone "they had to deal with," as they later admitted to me. Daniel would recover, and they learned that I would be someone they could count on to go to the mat to ensure that happened. I would be his advocate in all areas, including helping them to help him when necessary.

This mindset was not anything I was trained for. Instead, it was the realization of the obvious: it was up to the parents to be the difference in the well-being of our children, assuming the role of cheerleader and captain of our child's team, in school especially. We have become bold as individuals and as a community, fostering one of the biggest growths in understanding of this disorder that had little to do with medical convention. In fact we often butt heads with traditional medical practitioners who feel threatened by the progress of our children through the implementation of alternative treatments. Knowledgeable researchers, physicians, and practitioners have joined our ranks mainly because they became vested in the cause when their own child was diagnosed with autism.

The reaction from the school personnel did not surprise me as much as the reaction from other parents of children with autism. They often took my efforts and attitude as an affront to their interpretation of not only my child, but their own. They appeared to wonder why was I not accepting the conventional thinking that they had—the one dispensed by the traditional physician who had not studied autism in medical school. The mantra of "no hope, no cure" seemed to be the easiest one to accept for these parents, as opposed to "my child will recover from autism." To them and others, I was crazy to even think that recovery from autism was possible. But for those that also decided to find the answers for their children, something changed in them profoundly, as it did me. And it did so in ways that none of us would have imagined. Autism—and desperation for our children—changed us.

Over the years of mentoring parents, I found that there were core character attributes that seemed to make a difference in how a parent processed through grief, and how they managed to declare victory over autism too. These attributes were *tenacity, audacity, optimism, fearlessness, inquisitiveness, intuitiveness,* and *assertiveness.* It appeared that these attributes either were second nature to the parent of the child with autism, or the parent developed these traits. Many of them went on to help their children fully recover too, and others had children who were greatly improved. The rest had a sense of doing all they could to help their child medically despite having cycled back to acceptance as they got their child ready for a group home and adult services.

We had all gone through a level of battle that left us as bruised warriors, but not beaten.

Admittedly, I came into the community of autism parents with many of the seven attributes just as part of my personality makeup. But even with those underlying qualities already present, they had to be hewn into a form of action if the declaration of my son's full recovery was going to happen. What burned inside me was the "when" the recovery would happen; the "if" was non-existent. When I began to mentor families, it was surprising how many adults needed to be coached on setting boundaries, creating goals, and focusing on the possibilities rather than heading down the path of zero hope. I wondered at times if any of them had ever been in a business situation where all seven of the attributes would be demanded of them if they were to achieve success in their career. Oddly enough, I had conversations with a few CEOs and high-level executives who had to be coached through elements of these attributes to understand that their role as a parent was to be the CEO of their child, and that they had to make decisions to benefit the "company's" growth!

There is no one attribute that is more important than the others. They are all equal, except that at times, one or more will be called upon at higher levels. For instance, if you need to do some research, then you are tapping into *tenacity*, *inquisitiveness*, and *intuitiveness*. Need to get ready for an IEP meeting? Then you are potentially utilizing *audacity*, *fearlessness*, and *assertiveness*. When you head into a physician's office, chances are you are using all seven attributes, especially *optimism*.

What follows is a breakdown of each attribute, how it manifests in our quest for victory over autism, and how we develop each characteristic.

Tenacity

Think back to a time in your life when you wanted something so badly that you could picture the feeling of achieving it. Capture that thought and crystallize the impression in your mind. Was it a new car, a new house, a job opportunity, or even a relationship with someone significant? You dreamed about it, made plans, and knew that the object of your desire was yours if you just stuck with it. Heck, for many of you it was just sticking it out long enough to graduate from college.

In my days of working in a corporate office for a large retail company, I was put in charge of a fundraising effort for a local cancer institute, one that the whole industry supported. It was a high-profile undertaking, and there was the sense that if we raised enough money, someone's life would be saved. (Okay, that is sort of the whole purpose of every illness fundraiser.) But something about this campaign solidified into "saving someone's life," and the tenacious energy necessary to pull off this project got kicked into high gear, as did many of the other attributes.

On top of the usual pledge drive, it was decided that a simple baseball game between my company and a rival retailer would be put together with the buyers from both companies as the players. We brought in the presidents of both companies to act as umpires and then had a relief pitcher from the local major baseball team come to throw out the first pitch, had t-shirts made, encouraged the fans to come out, and in all other ways create a sense of fun energy around the event. What we initially thought would raise around $1,200 for a casual pickup baseball game turned into an over-the-top event where we raised around $267,000, with a thousand "fans" in attendance. My company lost the game, but we all had fun, raised a heck of a lot of money, and I was flown to Chicago for an industry dinner to be thanked for the fundraising effort.

The point of where this leads back to autism is that the tenacity to create the fundraising momentum led to an outcome that no one could have imagined. Likewise, the tenacity needed to help our children and family overcome the impact of autism happens at a sustained level over a period of time, for a possible outcome that no one could have imagined. The stakes are higher, and the need for tenacity is paramount to ensure success. You have had tenacity at other times in your life when it mattered most. Think of your days as an athlete and the level of dedication it took to stick with the practice schedule in a determined and resilient manner. Now it's your child's turn to receive that same level of tenacity, "stick-to-itiveness," if you will.

There is an understanding that autism is a marathon and not a sprint. It's very true, no matter how overused the saying is. Yet, too many of the families I meet want marathon results in sprint-level effort and time. They often declare that some diet or treatment did not work for their child after only a cursory effort on their part. And their tenacity to find what does work waxes and wanes with the thought that results should have been instantaneous. No, triumphing over autism requires tenacity—over and over.

For me, the tenacious tendency played out the most when I had to secure my son's first Individual Education Plan (IEP). I knew exactly what it was going to take for him to succeed and had everything lined up to ensure he received it, which he did. I was tenacious (bordering on obsessive) with the letter writing, meeting with everyone on the team in advance (at my insistence), and in creating a sense of energy around the effort. I was not giving up, even when the district initially said no. I dug in even further and came out of it with a secure plan in place. This is discussed further in chapter 4.

You may think that it was a lucky effort and that there's no way in the world your district would ever meet your child's needs, and you may be correct. But I also wonder how often the parents just give up because they are sick and tired of the battle. I totally understand why that would happen. But let me illustrate another situation that seemed impossible.

I began to volunteer as a special education advocate for children in the Department of Children and Families (DCF) here in my home state. The DCF allows for outside advocates to come in to help with the kids in their care because they are the most marginalized, especially educationally. I was called by the organization in charge of assigning advocates and asked what type of child I would like to represent. Without hesitation I asked them to give me a hard case, the kid that needed it the most. I was assigned a child who was indeed complicated. Kicked out of multiple foster care homes due to violent behavior, this eight-year-old boy's situation broke my heart. I was going to be his best advocate, almost as though his life depended on it, because in some ways it really did. I began to meet with those who were in regular contact with the child and pored over his evaluations, school reports, and other court files that documented the neglect and abuse he had suffered. This kid's life had been a mess, a testament to what no kid should ever have to go through.

He needed help, and the local school district, a large inner-city district, was not used to seeing advocates for the DCF kids advocating as much as I did for this boy. It was the content of the letters, the extent of my knowledge about the law, and the documentation of how each school district option was failing this child. I was also carefully lining up the need to move him out of district to a full-time residential placement. When the time came to have the child placed in an out-of-district school, I was sent to evaluate each option, but the one I had in mind for this boy was pricey. The cheaper one that the DCF wanted to put him in was a mess. It was a former women's prison, and looked like it. There was no way this facility would be able to serve this child, so I called the local DCF supervisor and notified them that I would not be signing any IEP with this place listed on it. I asked if they would allow me to review other placement options, but they had nothing further for me to look at and the next IEP meeting was a week away.

The next day, I was called by a supervisor from DCF who decided to barrel into me by saying that they were not going to pay for residential placement if the district would not do their share of splitting the cost. Seriously? She dared to confront me with a monetary concern when this kid needed help? She clearly had no idea who she was dealing with, how IEPs worked, or anything about what this child needed. How in the world did she end up in a profession meant to help children? Every ounce of constraint disappeared and I unleashed on the supervisor, letting her know that what she was suggesting did not belong in an IEP meeting and if she intended to get in my way, then DO NOT SHOW UP at the meeting. By the end of the conversation I was using choice words and eventually hung up (I was also eight months pregnant at the time, so she became fair game to hormones on top of the insult). And we needed to move fast to get him placed before I went on maternity leave.

She chose to not show up at the IEP meeting and resigned the child to another worker in order to not have any further dealings with me, which was perfectly fine. I walked into the meeting and they had the IEP filled out with the pricey option as the placement. The meeting was brief and cordial, and we walked out knowing it was the right thing to do for this boy. I continued for the next two years as this boy's advocate, ending only when he was adopted along with his twin brother. They were featured on a local news station that does segments on the kids that need to be adopted. The station reported that they received over a hundred calls to adopt the boys.

The point of this anecdote was the level of tenacity it took to stick with what was right. It was not unlike the level of tenacity for my own son. This is what I try to instill in parents as they begin to find the answers for their child. It is a sustained effort over a long period of time. And it is all worth it.

Audacity

The characteristic of audacity conjures up images of someone who is either way too pushy, a risk taker, or says the things the rest of us are thinking but we do not have the courage to say ourselves. Audacity is a necessary attribute in the journey to help our kids and family. This is also the one attribute I have to talk parents into the most. There is a sense with many of them that they don't want to "step on toes" or risk that someone will take it out on their child if they become too audacious and bold. They fear some sort of retribution. Note that the word *fear* is present in describing the reluctance to incorporate audacity as an attribute. There is *fear* of what others may think, *fear* of how they will handle themselves when forced into a characteristic that is foreign to them. And there is *fear* that once they head down this path they may never go back to how they once were, and they would be right.

Where this attribute comes up often is in conversations regarding IEP issues. Their child is not receiving appropriate services; the district is playing hardball and in all other ways not providing what the child needs. The parent is consumed with anxiety, doubt, worry, and anger over the situation, but declares they are helpless because the district has all the power. Nonsense.

As I coach these families, I make them aware of how to act respectful while still focusing on what the child needs. The key word is focus because it is in that paradigm of moving to the trait of audacity that we realize that it is incumbent upon us to act boldly when the need arises, especially when it comes to our child's educational needs.

One of my friends is the mother of two children on the spectrum, both in elementary school. As she approached a looming IEP meeting, she reached out and asked for a resource of a local special education advocate who would not charge exorbitant amounts. Knowing she had a long road ahead of her with both children, I volunteered to be the advocate, with the understanding that I would be showing her how to be the best advocate for her children going forward. Reading through the evaluations, it was apparent that the district had mislabeled one of her children as merely having behavioral issues, rather than those behaviors being a part of an overall autism diagnosis. I had a discussion with the mother on the need to change their perception of the child and work to create a better IEP. Mom agreed, and the first IEP meeting we had with the team could not have gone better. It was agreed that an evaluation on possible dysgraphia (writing disorder) was relevant, a full-time aide was assigned, and we got down to the business of "doing the right thing" for her son. So far, so good.

Then we hit turbulence in the form of a child who had a meltdown in class and threw an eraser at the teacher. The mother received a phone call from the assistant principal at the school letting her know that the child would be forced to write an apology note to the teacher as discipline. They wanted the child with possible dysgraphia to *write* the note. When the mother called me to ask about this discipline, I was astounded. They are making him write a note?! This is a complete violation of Section 504 laws that protect against disciplining a child for something that is caused by the disability. In this case it was a suspected disability, but it was, in our eyes, still part of Section 504 laws that protect this child from this type of discipline.

When the mother called to protest the discipline, she was told there was no choice and that it would happen anyway. So we fired off a letter outlining the "lack of common sense" and illegality of the action on the part of the assistant principal and district. We then notified them they needed to stop all further discipline of this nature and consult with the mother prior to any and all corrective action going forward. Audacity was in order here.

We called an emergency team meeting to discuss the move on the part of the school. This time around, the team was less than cordial, fully entrenched in the culture of circling the wagons to protect themselves. They insisted they would still possibly use writing as a method of discipline in spite of the mother's protest that it was relevant to the child's disability and would adversely affect him. We pushed back and said that if they did we would file immediately with the Office of Civil Rights (OCR), which protects individuals who fall under Section 504 disability laws. It was not an idle threat. We meant it, and they knew it. We also knew that there was no chance they would ever attempt a reckless decision to test our resolve on this issue.

In the town next door, I was the chairperson for a group that filed a class action OCR claim for a violation of Section 504 laws that impacted all of the kids in town who received special education services. The claim cost the district a hefty legal bill, which is why districts in general flat-out avoid dealing with the OCR as much as possible. We were the first class-action claim that the OCR attorneys took on, catalyzing a bunch of parents angry enough to be a part of this audacious move. I hear occasional objections from parents who are not keen on rocking the boat with the school district, and I am left to remind them that anyone who ever made a difference in their own life, or the lives of others, had to rock the boat. In their case, they owed it to their child to become bold without becoming rude or obnoxious (minus the necessary pushback to knuckleheads).

It also takes a whole bunch of audacity to make decisions in general for our children. Will we be bold and pursue a more aggressive form of treatments and therapies, or wait for all of the double-blind placebo studies before we make a move? Or will we use the studies to deter us from making any decisions that might benefit our child?

I had a conversation with a mother recently who has twins on the spectrum. I casually mentioned dietary changes and the mother grew squeamish because she had "heard" that diets didn't work, and that was good enough for her. When I challenged her supposition, she said she heard this from a very reliable source—another mother who had tried and failed at implementing the diet for her child. Since she had arrived at this conclusion based on hearsay rather than her own research or experiences, it became clear to me that she was either stuck in some part of the grief cycle or had jumped to *acceptance*. I wanted to instill in her a measure of audacity to step away from her perspective and consider the possibility that diet might actually help her children. My quick rundown on the benefits of the diet and how easy it would be to try was met with resistance, evidenced by her body language, but I persisted. I'm not sure if my efforts made a difference, but I definitely planted a seed because if there is one thing I can be persuasive about, it is the need to provide our kids with a proper diet.

When I first began to mentor, I was a bit dogmatic about the need for diet changes to begin healing. But as some of these parents went on to have recovered or significantly improved kids, they would come back to thank me for being such a crazy woman (read: audacious personality). A mom I mentored long distance also had the tone in her voice that dietary intervention was going to be too much to handle. But, after a few emails and a conversation, she too opted to give it a try. Now she still thanks me for getting her started down the path of understanding how to help her son. Her Facebook posts of his successes in high school are tremendous satisfaction to watch. Now she remembers how my audacity led her to find her own. She is quite prolific with her posts on diet now, which is weird twist to irony.

Audacity takes many forms, and it is in the act of stepping out of our comfort zone that we begin the path to acquiring it.

Optimism

On this journey of meeting and helping families find answers for their child, I could almost peg the ones who would hang in there through thick and thin of the journey. They would say with all sincerity that their child would recover or would improve, and by golly they were going to be the ones to drive the bus. And everyone else had better get on board with the optimism they exuded, or else. Then there were the ones who would declare that a prospective treatment or therapy would probably not work with their kid, repeating it often enough to be an anthem and self-fulfilling. Those were the ones that made me sad because they carried no trace of optimism in their character, the proverbial Eyeore of autism parents, destined to find fault, criticize the efforts of other parents, and in all other ways assert themselves to be victims of their child's autism.

There was a local author who wrote a book about her family's journey through autism that left me feeling incredibly depressed because there was not an ounce of optimism—or a reason for hope—in the book. At all. So when a newspaper reporter contacted me for a review of the book as an autism advocate, I had to be honest. I could not recommend the book in good conscience because there was no hope in it. How could a parent new to the diagnosis for their child read the book and wonder if this was their path too? No, I had to part ways with the philosophy of the writer in spite of it being a heartfelt book of her family's ordeal.

The author of the book was incensed with my published comments and wrote a letter to the editor outlining how her book was about her family's plight and should have been regarded differently. But from my perspective, no one should ever be discouraged from finding what works for their family. And no one should ever take away hope. Ever.

Admittedly, optimism was a trait I lacked when Daniel was first diagnosed. We had to grapple with his behaviors and health issues before any ray of optimism could peek through. Before optimism, I had to go through all six of the stages of grief until arriving at *resolve,* and even then I had to really hunt down the reason to be optimistic when I had yet one more diarrhea diaper to change. But optimism did come in the guise of other parents who were inspiring me with their own reasons to hope. They were doing things that made a difference in their children, and I wanted to be like them. They refused to give up, kept plugging away with their research, and attended conferences and seminars, all of which in turn generated optimism in them.

One of those first ridiculously inspiring parents I met in the beginning of the journey was Kim, who exuded keen knowledge on all things biologically to do with autism. She was a biochemist and had two children on the spectrum who were close in age to Daniel. Together, we kept each other going, and in many ways she is the one person I can count as my mentor. As she spoke from her biochemist perspective and how it related to our children, I found myself engrossed in her words. You see, knowledge to me was optimism personified. The more I learned from parents like Kim the more I would be filled with a new direction of what to research for my son. And that led to more answers, which led to more optimism.

As I was writing this part of the chapter, a relative wrote to tell me some devastating medical news. With a quick check on what the diagnosis meant in her situation, I sent her information that pointed to other possibilities to use for a second opinion, and not to be discouraged. It's a habit for me to look for other avenues when a bleak outcome is given as the prognosis. I will gravitate always to the belief that the answers are out there.

This is a tough trait to instill in the parents who are naturally pessimistic. They tend to be the ones that declare that something is not going to work, or is too difficult, expensive, not worth their effort to try. Still, I believed that if they just started to look for the answers and started treatments of some kind, that the trait of optimism would eventually kick in as they saw positive changes in their child. Many times that is exactly what happened. Then there were the few, truly few, who were determined to forego optimism for reasons of their own, which is probably one of the reasons why so many kids end up in group homes at young ages.

A friend of mine worked at one of these homes for many years and witnessed how the kids were coming in younger and younger. She said many of the parents were worn out while others were not able to cope with the day-to-day care. She was certain that if they had someone like me or another parent mentor to show them the way, they would have found the answers for their children. She also said that there were a few who simply could not be bothered with the effort to raise a child with special needs. Those were the parents who broke her heart the most because of the impact on the children.

Instilling optimism in a parent carries with it the responsibility of encouraging the parent to take the first step to begin researching the answers, even if it is purchasing a book, attending a conference, or hooking up with another parent who is knowledgeable and optimistic on these issues. That was why many of us parents began to volunteer: to bring the next parent along. The truth is that for each parent who does take that leap there will be a child getting better on the other end.

Fearlessness

Many of my Facebook friends who are in my autism group have personas that reflect a certain badass quality. They are advocates fighting for their children, leading causes and meeting with politicians to change laws for the sake of our children and families. So much can be written about the heroes in our community but it would seriously require a whole other book (which is not a bad idea).

For the parent just beginning the journey, developing the trait of fearlessness is best brought about after processing through the grief stages and getting to the *resolve* part. Yes, some parents are naturally fearless "getouttatheway" kind of people, but in the course of helping our children, the trait of fearlessness takes the form of gathering research-oriented information coupled with following instinct and making a decision that involves moving forward. It also takes the form of speaking up for the sake of our children as well as insisting and pushing back on their behalf as well. It takes the form of standing up to the individuals who do not understand what you and your child are up against, yet continue to offer their judgments and opinions on what you and your family should do.

The thing is that many of us don't recognize the trait of fearlessness until we are faced with a sick child and have to start making decisions for their well-being. It's not just courage that we call up in these extraordinary circumstances, but the true grit of determination to overcome the odds. Most parents would not look back at the decisions they made and call them fearless, but just something they had to do at the moment. They would be correct, except that the ongoing decisions that parents in the autism community make can be made daily.

I am one of those in the type A personality category that has few problems speaking up, pushing back, and exuding confidence. But the one time Rich and I were faced with a real difficult decision of whether or not to implement IVIG on Daniel, my sense of fearlessness waned and I called my sister, who has a degree in virology, to come ask the pertinent questions to the doctor. She was the one who reassured me on the decision to move forward with starting IVIG, and I am forever grateful to her. Continuing with IVIG after insurance refused to pay for it took another level of fearlessness, especially for Rich. Knowing that Daniel's well-being was at stake, Rich went into high gear to find a way to pay for the treatments.

When I mentored parents, all I had to do to instill fearlessness in them was to challenge them to take the necessary steps. Was it research they needed to do? Or was it making an appointment with a therapist, physician, or someone else that would lead to them to build momentum on their path to developing the necessary trait of fearlessness? It is definitely synergistic. Movement begets movement, which leads to making more bold decisions. That was how fearlessness began. Funny how it resembles the other stages too. Movement leads to making decisions, which leads to more movement and then positive outcome.

Louise Habakus runs an online blog community called *Fearless Parent*, for which I have contributed an article on grief. *Fearless Parent* exemplifies this whole principle of grabbing a hold of that fearless part within ourselves. They describe their site this way: "*Fearless Parent* is an innovative online media platform that's ahead of the pulse for today's thinking parent. The site offers information, commentary, and original content through our blogs, radio show, and community-based programming. The reporting is provocative, honest, and hopeful."

These parents totally speak my language—provocative, honest, and hopeful. Bravo! There are now legions of parents who have gravitated to this kind of perspective over the "no hope, no cure" mantra they had originally been told by physicians and others. They have determined that they would become fearless in the wake of making decisions because their child *deserved that from them*.

Instilling fearlessness in the next parent begins again with processing through the six stages of the grief cycle first. Once they get to *resolve*, then the trick is to not jump so forcefully into fearlessness that the parent becomes reckless instead. That is where diligence in doing your research on all topics that pertain to your child becomes key. This is why the other traits must also be in play for fearlessness to have strength of purpose and validity.

As an example of how fearlessness can run amuck, a mom I mentored became so wound up with a sense of fearless decision making that she ended up heading in a dozen different directions, wearing herself and her child out in the process. She implemented one treatment or therapy while pursuing several other options simultaneously. It is very common in our community to have parents so overwhelmed with the choices that we think we need to do everything at once, which exhausts everyone and depletes our finances quicker. It may or may not help the child, but the point to this is that the decisions were not necessarily well thought out or put into holistic perspective of how much of a toll it would take on everyone to do everything at once. Truthfully, there were probably times when I was guilty of this same scenario until I dialed it back to put some teeth into the decisions by doing a little more research. That was when the real fearlessness took off and began to propel me forward to a better outcome for my son.

Inquisitiveness

On this journey, the biggest surprise has been parents, physicians, therapists, and others who simply do not know that kids are recovering from autism. I hear it over and over: "I never knew that was possible." But there have been numerous articles, books, news segments, and even a published study that demonstrates that children are indeed recovering. The first book that I ran across like this was Karyn Seroussi's book titled *Unraveling the Mystery of Autism and Pervasive Development Disorder*, which was first published in 1999, a year before we received Daniel's diagnosis. In it, Seroussi outlines her own metamorphosis as she began to look into finding ways to help her son. This led her to start dietary interventions, behavior therapies, and supplements that led to her son's recovery from autism back in the late nineties.

I remember reading in her book that she had been inspired by another book written by Catherine Maurice titled *Let Me Hear Your Voice: A Family's Triumph over Autism*, which to this day is considered one of the first books that demonstrated recovering from autism was a possibility. Maurice's book was first published in 1993, a time when the Lovaas method of behavior therapy was considered controversial. Today, it is mainstream therapy, but back then it was unusual. Yet, this therapy method is what Maurice did for her daughter, which eventually led to her recovery from autism.

So, is it desperation that finally drives a parent to wonder if recovery from autism is possible for their child too? When does the instinct of inquisitiveness kick in? Aren't parents, physicians, therapists, and others even a little bit curious as to what worked to help these children to recover? Or are they easily dismissive of someone else's accounts of what happened to their child simply because it did not fit into their view of possibilities? So many dichotomies here to examine, but suffice it to say that the fact that you are holding this book means that you are inquisitive enough to wonder if it is possible.

At an autism conference in San Diego, I was sitting next to my friend Lisa Ackerman during a presentation by one of the doctors. This particular presenter had so much new information that to take notes seemed virtually impossible, but not to Lisa. As I saw her make this comprehensive list of things she planned to research later, I was blown away by how much she had gathered in just this one talk. And this was on top of the other items she was going to research from other talks she had heard. Lisa is one of the most brilliant women I have met. As the founder of Talk About Curing Autism (TACA), she is owed more thanks from the autism community than we could ever express. The key to Lisa's drive is her natural inquisitive nature. She wants to know as much as possible about one treatment modality or another, on top of just the things our families in the community are facing daily.

Even in the early days of Daniel's diagnosis, the whole inquisitive trait was enhanced by the advent of the internet, which I perused daily. At times I was looking up articles and information or corresponding online through Yahoo groups. Now it has evolved into Facebook groups. This was on top of talking to the top doctors doing the actual research of what I was reading, and then to other parents and activists who were in the trenches making a difference in the well-being of our children.

If osmosis derived from just being a wallflower in the room was required, that was what I was going to do in order to be a sponge of knowledge.

One thing that always struck me as odd was when I was asked a question that could be easily answered by using an Internet search engine. I always provided the answer with links for the other person to follow up. But a part of me wondered if they were doing their own research and not just basing their decisions on the opinions of others.

Enhancing an inquisitive trait is often done with the right kind of motivation. On the one hand, researching a new cell phone plan seems to be a great motivator for some to become inquisitive and resourceful. But when it comes to understanding autism, these same parents fall short by accepting whatever someone else tells them to do, or what is possible. Inquisitiveness is imperative if real knowledge is going to be attained and eventually used to make decisions. Become curious to all of the possibilities, and explore every avenue that makes sense to you. Then watch the flood of information cascade into a whole new world of what might work for your child.

Intuitiveness

Okay, I am just going to put this out there in the form of an understatement: I am incredibly intuitive when it comes to our children with autism. Some of those closest to me are laughing now reading that statement because of how often I have used intuition to pick up on things they need to look into further for their children. Some call it a gift. I call it well-honed instincts based on lots and lots of experience from working with families.

Intuition is that gut instinct we all have. It's just a matter of how much we listen to it before doubt overwhelms us. Many of us have stories that are associated with feelings of guilt for not following our parental instinct. I have heard, over and over, "I knew it wasn't a good idea but the doctor said it was, so I went along with it." Or I have heard, "Against my better judgment, I signed the IEP."

Our intuition is the guiding light that our fundamental principles follow. We are guided intuitively, even to the people who cross our lives. We are particularly attuned to needs of our children. If something is just not right with them, we see and feel it intuitively.

When Daniel was a year old he received his MMR, varivax, and polio vaccines on the same day. The next day he had a 105 degree fever and diarrhea that would not be abated by traditional remedies. I called the doctor's office about the fever and diarrhea and was told that it was a normal reaction to the vaccines. But something told me this was not normal. Within two weeks, I took him back to the pediatrician's office to say something was just not right with him. He was crankier than usual and seemed to be in some sort of inexplicable pain, not to mention the persistent diarrhea. The doctor made a cursory suggestion to try crackers for the diarrhea and to "keep an eye" on how he is feeling because nothing told him anything was wrong.

Two weeks later we were back in his office with the same complaints, but no viable remedy was offered, even after another visit two weeks later. The only reason why the timing on this is clear is because we received the pediatrician's file on Daniel when we moved and had to change pediatricians. There were the doctor's notes with dates showing how often I came in with the same list of symptoms. I knew something was up, and there is a part of me that wonders if the doctor knew too, but it was not confirmed until a few months later when his physical therapist suggested we get him tested for autism spectrum disorder.

Heading into the milieu of the diagnosis, I didn't have a clue what it all meant for Daniel, but a measure of naiveté mixed with intuitiveness led me to simply say "Let's go fix this" to his physical therapist. And I repeated this often over the next few years, not knowing exactly where it came from. Only intuition had me on a course to find the answers for Daniel.

When I would mentor parents on the principle of using their intuition to make decisions, it often involved the concept of a "leap of faith" based on what they felt was the right thing to do versus what others were telling them to do. And at times that was a huge caveat for those who were used to operating strictly from their head and not their gut. The neurologist I mentioned earlier is one who relied on her medical training to make a decision, foregoing any input from a mother's intuition. Simply put, relegating the intuition as irrelevant means that some decisions do not get made largely due to fear of the unknown.

Intuition means simply listening to the gut, especially when instinct is moving you in one or another direction. It's a repeated thought, or an opportunity dropped in your lap to just make an appointment with a specialist or implement a remedy for your child.

Intuition is also what can stop us from heading in the wrong direction. When Daniel was at his worst, around the age of two, it was suggested by a friend that I take him to a healer who used crystals for healing. It was against every ounce of intuition that crystals were the way to go for Daniel, but I went forward with it because I didn't have any ideas where else to turn. Arriving at this small office, we are told the appointment was going to cost four hundred dollars out of pocket. Gulping at yet one more expensive appointment, I hung in there just in case it was something I was just freaked out about because I didn't understand it. When the wait for the therapist went to over ninety minutes, I took that as a sign that we were simply not meant to be there. It doesn't mean that this modality has not helped other children, because I truthfully don't know. But I knew that it was not meant for Daniel, and I left the office.

Intuition kicks in heavily too, when it comes to protecting our children from harm. I met a mom whose daughter was assaulted at school. While the daughter was nonverbal, there were certain changes in the daughter's behavior that led the mother to challenge the school with her belief that something happened at school. It was later determined that an aide in the class had pushed the child to the floor. Sadly, this is not an isolated incident, and our non-verbal children are the most likely to be hurt.

In my days in a corporate environment there was a tremendous need to base some decisions on instinct, including those I could trust with business decisions that reflected what was good of my company. It was that same sense of intuitiveness that kicked in at my son's first IEP meetings. I would observe body language, listen for contextual changes in the flow of the meeting, and in all ways get a feel for the people in the room. I understand that it's not everyone who does, but many parents (who have this same business sense) need to realize that it is entirely applicable in all things related to their child, especially when working with those individuals making the decisions that will impact their child. One of those parents was a large-business owner who had to be convinced to bring his business savvy to the IEP meeting. He was certain that the school district would simply take care of his son if he was nice enough to them, so he insisted on bringing cookies to the IEP meeting (something I discourage, for a number of reasons).

I heard from this father several months later, and he was bitterly discouraged by his experience with the district, lamenting the thought that cookies would seal the IEP deal better than using his business instincts to represent his son. He switched gears pretty quickly after that.

Assertiveness

It isn't a stretch to realize that I came to the autism table with the trait of *assertiveness* firmly in place. But there were still areas where I didn't realize that assertiveness was in order because I never had to use that trait in some situations before, especially in a doctor's office or over the phone with an insurance company. In some ways, the trait of assertiveness overlaps with the trait of audacity, except that assertiveness requires speaking up and audacity requires making bold decisions. That's why they make great partners in a variety of situations.

I have a few friends who are naturally assertive. They can walk into a room and command attention just by being there. And then there are other friends who want absolutely no attention brought to themselves so they keep quiet to avoid rocking the boat or having someone think badly of them.

We all have our boundaries, and we need to defend them when someone encroaches on our efforts to help our children and our families get through the worst of days with autism. For some, it is necessary to assert themselves with physicians, therapists, school districts, and even other family members if they are to survive with their sanity intact. If you even think that avoiding this trait of being assertive is going to help you with your child, you are completely wrong. If you are not assertive on this journey, by speaking up for your child and the well-being of your family, then you are not doing your job. Period. I cannot say this more emphatically and will not sugarcoat what is necessary. It is incumbent upon you as parents to overcome autism with the help of assertiveness, chutzpah, cojones, wherewithal, confidently persuasive, or whatever you want to call it, as long as it means the same thing.

In his book, *When I Say No, I Feel Guilty: How to Cope—Using the Skills of Systematic Assertive Therapy*, clinical-experimental psychologist Manuel J. Smith, PhD, declared a bill of assertive rights for those who have a problem with setting boundaries.

A BILL OF ASSERTIVE RIGHTS

I: You have the right to judge your own behavior, thoughts, and emotions, and to take the responsibility for their initiation and consequences upon yourself.

II: You have the right to offer no reasons or excuses for justifying your behavior.

III: You have the right to judge if you are responsible for finding solutions to other people's problems.

IV: You have the right to change your mind.

V: You have the right to make mistakes—and be responsible for them.

VI: You have the right to say, "I don't know."

VII: You have the right to be independent of the goodwill of others before coping with them.

VIII: You have the right to be illogical in making decisions.

IX: You have the right to say, "I don't understand."

X: You have the right to say, "I don't care."

You have the right to say no, without feeling guilty.

I especially like the last line the most since it is usually the one many of us choose as a last resort when we have nothing left to give. I will discuss that one part more in detail in chapter 5 on marriage and chapter 7 about care for the caregiver.

As the trait of assertiveness pertains to your child, it is a mixture of sticking to your guns on what is right mixed with coping skills on getting through the worst of days we all have to endure. It is speaking up to any and all individuals connected to our children, and even speaking up at times to our children and setting boundaries with them if they are able to understand. I used to say that I give a thumbnail of excuse for my son's behaviors related to autism, and the rest of it he needed to comply with for safety's sake (again, every child is different in their ability to understand). It's easier to enforce this when a child is younger than when they become larger and more difficult to manage.

I will discuss further, through much of the rest of this book, where the trait of assertiveness was necessary and how it catapulted us and others to declare victory over autism too.

Chapter Three

Who Cares What Anyone Else Thinks?!
Live by Your Own Truth and Opinions

"I was told that there is no hope for my child. They say that he will probably end up in a group home or something," said the anguished mother who had called me early on a weekend morning. Calmly, but with firmness, I had to convince this mother that she had just been handed a load of bull. "The physician is wrong and you are about to prove it," I replied. "Never accept this kind of crap from anyone again!" And the mentoring began, coaxing this mother to understand that it was necessary to be assertive, even a little bitchy, when it came to the well-being of her child.

But with every phone call from a beaten-down parent, I had to ask what made the difference between those who overcame the negative declarations from others and those who allowed someone else's adverse opinion to become their truth too. Why did some adopt elements of the seven core attributes while others did not? What principles did they live by, if not their own? We all need personal guiding principles to stabilize our core belief system. Add autism to whatever guiding principles we adopt, and there is a whole different perspective on what we will accept as our truth.

Developing these core-strengthening principles became an essential part of mentoring to instill in the parents the resolve they would need, and the courage that would come along the way. These principles *work*, and have helped to shift the mindset of many other parents on the journey toward wellness for their child. They also fall in line with the stages of grief and the essential attributes of the bold parent. Much of it appears sort of redundant in theme, except there are layers of understanding in each of these chapters. And maybe you can add your own core truths that would reverberate. The purpose in this portion is how we strive to adopt the essential traits of the bold parent into our daily lives as challenged parents of special children.

Find Out What It Is You Do Not Know (Yet)

This principle falls in line primarily with the trait of inquisitiveness. What is it you do not know or understand? How often did I suggest to a parent to get educated on one thing or another and not just take my word for it. Parents getting educated is crucial and the cornerstone of the recovery process. That is the caveat then. How does a parent determine who, what, where, and how to get educated? The when part is a given—right now! Although I sincerely believe most parents would do anything to find the answers for their child if they just knew where to start.

Like most parents in our community, I became an expert at using search engines and online groups, taking advantage of conferences and seminars, and finding the right people to talk to that would raise my level of understanding and awareness. It was serendipitous that I would be led to the answers just by virtue of the fact that I was looking for them. In 2002 I happened to attend the DAN conference in San Diego. DAN stood for Defeat Autism Now, a part of the Autism Research Institute which was started by Dr. Bernard Rimland, long regarded as the pioneer of the idea that children with autism could be treated and recover. At the conference, I happened to stumble on a hallway conversation between one of the presenters and a small group of parents. This group had gathered to speak with this leading researcher after hearing his presentation on how the age of insult to the immune system (meaning, the age when the immune system is triggered to go haywire), mixed with genetics, determined what type of disorder or disease an individual could potentially get. The researcher gave several examples of how the age of the person was relevant to how the developing brain responded to the immune system insult. He showed a rising trend in autism being identified at the age of around four, followed by the rise in children diagnosed with attention deficit disorder (ADD) or attention-deficit/hyperactivity disorder (ADHD) at around the age of seven, and then obsessive-compulsive disorder (OCD) and anxiety disorders around the age of ten. It culminated with an uptick in teenage mental health disorders, followed by a rise in adult-onset autoimmune disorders as the rise in immune triggers continued.

It was an eye opener to many of us in the room, and I began to connect the dots of all of the illnesses in my family members and what possibly could have been the trigger to their immune system that set off the downward spiral. We obviously had our genetic predisposition gun loaded, so it was when (or if) we had an immune system trigger that would set in motion a potential health challenge.

In my family, we have a long list of ailments, including substance abuse, mental health disorders, cancer, gastrointestinal autoimmune disorders, skin problems, and other health issues. Most of our families in the autism community have this dynamic in their own gene pool too. But what is it that predisposes one family over the other? And what sets the trigger in motion in the individual? These were the questions I wondered, which is why I was glad to see this same presenter in the hallway.

As he continued to answer questions, I had my chance and asked, "You mention the age of insult to the immune system. My own (relative) received nine vaccines on the same day when he was nineteen and heading into the Army. When he got out two and half years later he had developed severe gastrointestinal issues, followed by mental health issues. While still in his twenties he was diagnosed with a heart condition that has been linked to mercury toxicity. At the age of thirty-eight he had a heart attack. Today he is not a fully functioning adult. If he had received the same number of vaccines as my son had, would my (relative) have had autism too?"

Without hesitation the researcher said yes, and with such emphasis that there was no doubt of his certainty. His emphatic response explained a lot about my family's long list of generational health conditions, and why my son was born with the same genetic predisposition but experienced the environmental trigger sooner. This little revelation learned in the hallway at a conference spurred a research frenzy when I got home, leading me to realize we were looking at a catastrophe in the illnesses our generation of children were about to experience. Sadly that prediction was more than accurate and we began to see disorders that never existed when my generation was children.

A couple of years later, I was asked to participate in a series of radio interviews alongside researchers and physicians who were treating our children. One of those physicians was Dr. Anju Usman, who is revered in our community as a dedicated, passionate physician who truly understands how to help our children. When we were on the radio—me in California and Dr. Usman in Chicago—the radio interviewer asked about the escalating numbers of autism and what it meant. Something about the conversation with the researcher in San Diego came back and I outlined the prediction that the children with autism were the canaries in the mine signaling the problems that are going to follow.

I went on to repeat much of what the doctor said at the conference in San Diego, beginning with the rise in autism, followed by the rise in ADD, ADHD, and OCD, which leads to teen mental health issues and the comorbidities like depression, obesity, and behavior problems that follow kids when they are put on medication or left to deal with their issues through substance abuse and risky behaviors. Next up would be an increase in autoimmune disorders in the late teens and early twenties (college years). I opined then that the next major epidemics we would be hearing about would be multiple sclerosis (MS) and amyotrophic lateral sclerosis (ALS).

Dr. Usman chimed in after this litany and said, "She's absolutely right." She added greater understanding on why this is so with the right environmental influences. Ten years later, and our radio conversation began to look like a fortune telling session. Only thing is the teen mental health disorders were escalating at a faster rate than any of us imagined, with new terms like pediatric autoimmune neuropsychiatric disorder associated with strep (PANDAS) and pediatric acute-onset neuropsychiatric syndrome (PANS), Tourettes, and generalized anxiety disorder coming into our vernacular. The thing I also realized was how much those parents needed information for their children as well. Some of these were typical kids one day, and in a mental health crisis the next. Pharmaceutical remedies are the natural choice for physicians to recommend because that is all they know. So reaching these parents to engage in the process of finding answers became the next battle cry.

I happened to host Beth Alison Mahoney, Esq., as a guest at a TACA Massachusetts meeting. Beth is the author of the book *Saving Sammy*, which dealt with her then twelve-year-old son's descent into obsessive-compulsive disorder (OCD) after a strep infection. After repeated attempts to find answers through traditional medicine, Beth researched further and found a physician several states away who was using amoxicillin in higher doses to defeat the kind of strep her son had, which had led to his mental health breakdown. While Beth's son was victorious and went on to be a successful adult, there were many other parents and kids going through the same nightmare. Beth is now a crusader for this next battle, and she became that when she got herself educated on what she didn't know.

When in Doubt, Go with What *Feels* Right

Parents are not taught to trust their "gut instinct" in decision making, and a completely cerebral (and often misguided) method gets ingrained. This is obviously the area that deals with the trait of intuitiveness. It can also invoke assertiveness in great measure too. In the previous chapter, I gave examples of how the intuitive trait plays out. In this section of discussing "doubt" there has be an understanding that much of the doubt will come in the early stages of the grief cycle as a parent struggles with their child's needs, their own emotions, and all of the stress that it includes.

At times, there is a leap of faith and then there is a jump across the chasm of faith that is necessary when making a decision. For some it is taking a leap and choosing to homeschool, or try a new approach based on where their parental instinct is leading them. Of course, all of this involves research and discussing all available options, but a huge part involves just doing it because it feels right. The pushback from others comes in the form of those who believe they know more than you on what you need to be doing. Admittedly, those I have mentored may have at one time or another felt that way about me as I helped them navigate the intricacies of diet, treatments, and even school issues. Some would push back to let me know that their child or their family life was not able to cope with all I was suggesting, and they were probably correct. Bottom line is you need to trust your own instinct over the opinions of others—even others who have their own expertise to share. If it does not resonate with your family, then wait until it does or find something else.

I figured out quickly that if I relied upon the opinion of others, including physicians and experts, over my own instinct then I would be making a dreadful mistake. It was innate to follow that instinct, especially when it meant walking away from something or someone that was clearly not helpful, and potentially harmful. At one time, Daniel was a candidate for surgery to lengthen his heel cords since they were tight and would potentially affect growth of the bone or how his feet would position. He was starting to show signs of having a problem when he began to trip over his own feet on the soccer field. We took him to a number of orthopedic surgeons over the years and each one had a different opinion on the options, and each one was incredibly invasive. We decided to wait until he hit his teen growth spurt to see how much of an issue it would be. It turned out that the six inches he grew in one year had no impact on the bone growth or his ability to do activities. If we had chosen the more invasive option it could have presented with other side effects later. Instead of relying on the opinions of the physicians, we chose the path of "wait and see," and it turned out to be right for him.

Yes, being guarded in some of our decisions and sticking with them once they were made was not new. But we could have let the opinions of the physicians sway our decision, or the well-intended comments from family affect our mood. But we didn't. Speaking of family, that is the area where this principal of standing your ground is most necessary. A mom I mentored had difficulty in her marriage because her husband tended to side with the judging, meddling members of his family over his own wife in the decisions being made to help their children. Since she was the one home with them she implemented dietary changes to see if it would modulate their health and behavior. When it did by a large measure, she went to extraordinary lengths to protect them from coming in contact with the foods that they could not eat. But the in-laws were determined to undermine her effort by providing the children junky foods and treats, even plying the children with it at family events. The mother needed an ally in her husband, not an adversary.

So she stuck to her commitment to forge a way to better health in her son and daughter, even sending an email to the family members letting them know of her intent to keep her children away from the foods and that she needed their support in the effort. This won her huge respect from the in-laws, and they agreed to no longer serve the children the offending food. Personally, I think the email should have come from her husband, but that is a whole other topic to be discussed in chapter 5.

You Know More Than You Think You Do

I attended a presentation on autism treatments from a local pediatric neurologist, one who headed up the whole pediatric neurology department at a hospital. He was a sincere, genuinely caring physician who said he approached autism like he wished other doctors had treated his mother when he was growing up. This doctor went on to explain how his mother was abused verbally by the doctors she came to for help for his special needs sister. As a physician, he said he wanted to validate and listen to families, not disparage them. That's how he ended up in neurology, eventually helping autism families.

As he lined up the treatment information and studies in his lengthy list of slides, I was puzzled at the redundancy from what most of us in the room already knew. We had been breathing this information for the past decade, so it was perplexing why different information was not presented. Then he said, "Everything I know about autism I learned from the parents." Aha. Yes, indeed he had. This explained why the information he was presenting was not new: we had been his teachers.

This is where the traits of tenacity, audacity, and intuitiveness come in to play. I am one of many parents who end up educating physicians and therapists in the course of a visit with them. Maybe we can't help it, or maybe it's just that the discussion segues into an area where we are very knowledgeable. On many occasions the conversation completely evolves to be about them and what is going on with their family. I then pass along information they may find helpful.

There have also been the conversations with total strangers that begin with a simple comment. When I head down the path of sharing information, I find out that I am speaking with a physician, lawyer, therapist, or some other expert. You see, I learned long ago that parents truly do know more than they think they do, and they need to rise to the occasion of believing this about themselves too. If you follow the rest of the mantras of finding out what you don't know, trusting your instincts, setting boundaries, etc., then trusting that you know more than you think you do should follow. With the right traits of the bold parent, it is inevitable that you too will be the expert in all things to do with your child's needs.

Several of my friends are teachers, so when they gave me behind-the-scenes feedback on what the districts think about parents who have a child receiving school services, I paid attention to what they had to say. Not only did they give good advice on how to handle Daniel's educational needs, but they also let me in on how the IEP team perceived my actions. Most of the time it was positive, and other times there was a dividing line between the district's priorities and mine. No matter; I knew more than they did about the child I was representing: my son. I knew he was capable of so much more and would achieve developmental skills with the right motivation. I was also banking on him one day not needing special education or interventions of any kind and reminded them that their objective should be to graduate him out of services because he had achieved all benchmarks and goals; not that he was squeezed through the one-size-fits-all system.

When a friend opted to follow an aggressive diet and bio-medical protocol for her son with mental health disorders (not autism), she knew that the psych meds were not the answer for him. Her further research led her to have such a strong understanding of her son's conditions that she could recite studies on various treatments that had a direct benefit to her son. She became well-rounded enough in conversations that she often had to educate the physicians, enough to excite the physicians to study from the copious research she had been doing, complete with MRI's to prove how the therapies impacted her son's brain.

When I speak with other proactive parents as a group, I am often astounded to discover that their knowledge level on the latest treatments and therapies is miles ahead of mine. I can keep up on the vernacular and general information, but their expertise often far surpasses my own. I am then their student, and gladly so. It is common for my local autism group to host various speakers, including education leaders, physicians, therapists, authors, and those who are renowned in their field. We occasionally invite them to lunch or dinner just to extend our visit and encourage a more private conversation. What often happens, however, is that the parents end up educating the expert, even in their own field.

As parents, we are so resolute that we become the driving force behind developing our understanding and knowledge base (including research physicians who happen to be parents of children with autism). We have become the experts, and we are flat out shocked that traditional medicine practitioners are behind. This is why we cannot always defer to a medical practitioner or therapist. It's okay to investigate something further. It is not okay to assume that your knowledge base is irrelevant. It's not. You know more than you think you do.

Don't Be Afraid to Ask Questions . . . Especially "Why?"

This is a section of the book that follows the traits of inquisitiveness and assertiveness. Maybe a few of the others too, like audacity and tenacity, similar to the three-year-old child who has to ask "why" questions repetitively. Okay, maybe not that incessantly, but you get the picture. Ask, as a matter of habit, why one practice, protocol, treatment, placement, or whatever is necessary or the best option.

During IEP meetings, I would often ask each team member separately why they believed a particular recommendation was necessary, or asked for their opinion in some other way. It built rapport and promoted collaboration among the team. Oddly enough, I later met Dr. Vaughn Lauer, PhD, who wrote in his book *When the School District Says No . . . How to Get to the Yes!* how asking questions of the team is part of the process of a good outcome. It doesn't always mean you are going to get the answer you want, just that you want someone to elaborate on an opinion or a decision that will affect your child.

When it was determined that Daniel no longer qualified for an IEP or Section 504 at the end of his high school freshman year, I listened and asked the obvious question of why they believed a removal from Section 504 protection would help him succeed in the classroom. They then outlined how a general education plan would work to provide what he needed since he was choosing to ignore some of the accommodations set up for him in the 504. Yes, my son was avoiding anything that looked like an accommodation to help him in the classroom.

Why I was not told this sooner was bothersome, but I also took a step back and decided to see how far he would go without educational protection in place. He was on the honor roll and doing well while ignoring the accommodations in place. I wondered how far he would go without them. So I agreed to remove him from the 504, but would put the whole thing on a short leash if the accommodations became necessary again. In fact, he did very well that year. And it all began with the question long ago of *why*.

The second favorite question to ask is *why not*. I say that because when I would see snippets of stories on children recovering from autism, I dared to wonder *why not* my son. When I wrote our story of recovery for *Mothering* magazine in 2004, I heard from a flurry of parents from all over the world who asked the same question of *why not* their child too.

Perhaps owing to impatience, the questions were constant in the quest for Daniel's return to health and well-being. I did a lot of research, of course, but the asking questions part seemed intuitive to do too. Just as parents educated the experts on what was working for our children, we are in a continuous mode of educating each other. What is working for one parent might be worth looking into for another parent in attendance. It is not unusual for us to share so much information that we wind up meeting for several hours at a stretch.

I used to bring small notepads to group meetings. Those in attendance probably would have recorded some of our sessions if not for the noisy background. I also found that some online groups had an astounding understanding of complex information. And all of us began by simply asking questions.

No One Knows the Potential of Any Child, Especially Yours! Ignore the Limitations Imposed by Others

There is nothing worse than hearing the words "Your child has autism spectrum disorder," followed by the words "will probably end up in a group home one day." We are one of many who received this pronouncement from the diagnosing physician— and many others along the way—of what the future held for our child. None of it painted even a measure of hope. Today, of course, Daniel has defied medical expectations. When he was born, we were told that he would probably not be able to be an athlete because of his club foot. Instead, he went on to be on his high school cross country and track team. We were told he may not talk or live a normal life, but I often tell parents that now he won't shut up and he is so normal that he is grounded until he leaves for college. That kind of normal.

Our children are assigned all kinds of labels, with accompanying predictions of the kind of life they will live. Pick a label like ADHD and the image of medications, behavior problems, and potential problems as an adult are conjured up. With autism spectrum's wide definition, the label simply does not fit a particular pattern, and no one knows about the child in front of you quite like you. So raise the bar high and give them the encouragement and support to follow the raised expectations of what they can achieve. This is probably why I don't use the term "autistic" to define children with autism. To me, it appears that the label of autism is synonymous with the child. It's the same reason why I don't use the term diabetic, asthmatic, or allergic but rather a child (person) with the disorder, syndrome, or illness. I'm not trying to be politically correct, just more accurate.

I was in an IEP meeting and the school psychologist declared the child fit the criteria for "mentally retarded" (an egregious term), which immediately caused the mother to burst into tears. I told the psychologist that nowhere in any of the medical reports is the term *mentally retarded*. Further, we suggested that one of the reasons this fourth grade child could not read might have something to do with an undiagnosed visual perception disorder.

The look on the faces of those in the room signaled that they may have missed something in their evaluations of the child. They shuffled through the reports, nodded heads, and finally agreed there was more to consider on why the child faced so many academic challenges. Soon after, the parents took their child to a behavioral optometrist who later confirmed a significant vision processing disorder, which was helped with prism lenses and therapy. Had the parents bought into the predetermined label, they might not have looked further and the school would have lowered the child's benchmarks for achievement.

At another IEP meeting, I was the advocate for a middle school boy who had been assigned a court-appointed lawyer to attend the meeting because the boy was getting into trouble at school often, earning the label "troublemaker." As I read through the reports and evaluations, I noticed a pattern of an undiagnosed educational disorder that left the boy unable to read or write, passed to the next grade every year in spite of his lack of academic progress.

The behavior therapist at the school decided to create yet another behavior modification plan, and I asked that she not speak until we addressed the very serious issue of the child's academic problems that could be causing his behaviors at school. As she attempted to ignore the request, I pointed out to the rest of the team that the boy could not read or write. The attorney was shocked at this apparent oversight in the court documents, expressing dismay that the school was not fully addressing his academic issues, only his behaviors.

As the tearful single mother sat beside me, I began to get a picture of how the labels had probably followed this child for a very long time: single mother, low-income household, academically struggling overweight teenager who ended up bullying others to get his way. Every single bit of his history spelled "troublemaker." I turned to the mother and said, "How did you let this happen?" Truthfully, I knew how. She had adopted the labels, for herself and for her son.

This is why the labels are only meant to be a springboard to finding the way past the odds. I think one of the best examples of overcoming the labels was a picture on my Facebook of an expensive, delicious looking lobster meal, with the caption: "Take that, guidance counselor!" We need to take that same sentiment and apply it to our children. No one knows their potential, so let's just decide that it is limitless.

You Are *Always* the Captain of Your Child's "Team"

Nothing irritates me more than hearing a school administrator refer to the "team" in such a way that the parent believes they are not a part of the team, but an outsider on the opposite side of the table. I sat in an IEP meeting representing another child when the chairperson said, "The team has agreed that the child does not qualify for extended year services."

I was astounded, and said, "Excuse me, but we are a part of the team too, and we are not in agreement. So if you want to say that the district staff has 'determined,' that would be more accurate. Otherwise," I continued as I pointed at the mother and me, "we are a part of this team and are not in agreement. We believe she does need extended year services." The chairperson stammered her clarification, but it was still like nails on chalkboard. *Stop it*, already.

The mother had assumed a high profile with the district because she realized that, as a parent of a child with special needs, she had to be fully in charge of the process, meaning she had a clear picture of what her role was as her child's parent and advocate. I was the advocate who just happened to come along for added support. The district, like many others, was in the habit of condescending to parents or in some way marginalizing their role. Some will patronize with their tone or body language or become caustic in an effort to undermine the parents; or perhaps it is just the culture of the school or district. Parents can also act unreasonable and unprofessional, making the whole notion of a team effort irrelevant because the IEP meetings have become habitually acrimonious. So much can be said on this part that I will leave it for chapter 4.

But I will say that unless a parent figures out quickly that they are the *captain* of the team, then they have given up that role to someone else. When I fully understood that I needed to be in charge of those around Daniel, it came with the understanding that I would do anything needed to help him succeed. I also had high expectations of others too. As mentioned before, I wrote letters, made requests, made sure he was on time for appointments, and always came prepared to meetings.

If the district staff, therapists, and others serving my son had an opinion, I listened. I also expected the same of others, and it worked. But the persona I developed in this role was more like King Arthur and the Knights of the Round Table. While we all had an equal voice in the dialogue, I took on the part of leading the discussion by asking relevant questions or expressing concerns. My intuition was in high gear as I absorbed all they had to say in order to make decisions for his well-being. It's not rocket science, just common sense and a whole lot of chutzpah to assume the captain role at all times. If the captain role does not suit you yet because you are still trying to process through grief, then give it some time. Just know that there will need to be a time that you will be required to step it up.

I totally understand how a parent needs to process through the grief cycle and come to the captain role of their own accord. It's a mixture of confidence and outrage, in many respects, where the line in the sand becomes clearer and the direction of what you need to do to help your child becomes more certain. In chapter 5 we are going to discuss what happens when both parents jockey to be the child's captain with a desire to head in different directions.

You Matter Too

This mantra is possibly the hardest one for parents to accept. The care of our children, especially our children with special needs, trumps our own needs, even our own health. But the real

mantra is that when it comes to the autism family, everyone matters. I am the epitome of how this mantra was not followed. You
see, I didn't matter to me. And I think Rich felt the same way
about himself. Our focus was our children, as it should be, but as
we were both navigating the clutches of grief after the diagnosis,
we sort of lost sight of how we were letting go of ourselves. If
you ask a parent who is in high-gear mode to get their child well,
they will often tell you that they (as the parent) do not matter.
They don't care about anything other than the quest for whole-
ness of their child. All the while they are losing pieces of themselves, and they may not even know it.

It's a bad habit we get into when we shelve who we are
as individuals in favor of who we are as parents. It's not that
we choose one role or the other, but rather how we blend the
roles. What happens when a child is diagnosed is that we head
down the path of just trying to wrap our head around what the
diagnosis means, and how our lives will change as a result. I
could not have even fathomed the idea that I was supposed
to take care of myself alongside finding answers for my son.
Something had to give, and in my case it was sleep, proper
nutrition, and exercise. Chapter 7 speaks directly to what this
kind of tunnel vision cost me before I figured out that I had to
fill in the empty bucket of health—the bucket that seemed to
be filled with holes because my perspective on what mattered
was so skewed.

This is one of those mantras that needs to be repeated over
and over to each other as part of the parent community, and to
ourselves. You matter too. If this is not adopted to its fullest
extent, then we as parents fail to thrive over the long haul of
securing health and well-being for our child and our family. It's
that simple.

You Are Not Alone

It is the emails that I and others receive that have kept many of
us active in the autism community. We are the thread of hope
for the next generation, with the autism numbers skyrocketing
and traditional medicine still providing little or no answers. By
contrast, if the child had been diagnosed with cancer, diabetes,

asthma, or food allergies, there would have been a different approach to how the family was provided information. This is the arena of traditional medicine, so they know the route to advise parents on, and even where to receive parental support.

Autism is different. There are no answers yet in traditional medicine, and the support is even sparser. That is why autism organizations that support parents with information are crucial. I have received countless emails and phone calls, and occasionally a parent showing up at my doorstep looking for information. Mainly, they want to know that they are not alone in this journey. It's the parent who asks for help that later becomes the parent who reaches out to the next parent to help them through too.

I have no doubt that the uptick in murder/suicides in our community is linked to that feeling of being alone while fighting despair every step of the way. No one should feel alone, and it is up to the rest of us in the community to ensure they don't. Likewise, the parent of the child needs to reach out to find the community that resonates with them, either online or in person.

One of the best examples of how a group grew out of this notion that they needed support from each other is The Thinking Moms' Revolution. This group consists of parents who met online when they were all were drawn to the same treatment modalities, which led to a book about their individual efforts to treat their children from autism and spread the word that children were getting well. It was a synergistic bond that brought these parents together, helping them realize that they were not alone. Indeed, they would soon start something that would spread around the world. Many of these parents are my friends today. I just wish I had known them when our journey began, but am grateful that they are here today for the next generation of parents.

The Thinking Moms' Revolution

What began as a collective journey
Of stories around the globe
From Autism to recovery, and with whatever happens
in between
A tight-knit group of parents were drawn to support
each other

Traveling the Autism journey
While learning, identifying, laughing, crying,
celebrating—experiencing a full spectrum of life
and emotions
Creating a Revolution along the way
Not for the weak
Always with hope in sight
We walk together
And invite you to do the same.[1]

The Answers Are Out There for Your Child!

There are those who would surmise that because my son recovered that I believe other children can too. And they would be correct. But you have to know that even if my son were not recovered yet, I would still be searching for the answers because I am convinced they are out there for every child, every person, and every health issue.

For everything we have learned along this journey, I am humbled by how much we still don't know. We are not even scratching the surface of understanding how to beat the health impact of autism, let alone how to overcome autism entirely. So, every time I hear of a new treatment or therapy that is showing promise (in spite of naysayers who disregard anything to do with treating autism), I get excited because the treatment or therapy may help even one more child and family.

When I hear of a child that has received the diagnosis of ADD, ADHD, Aspergers, anxiety issues, OCD, Tourettes—or even a rare disorder—I am firmly in the camp that the answers are not hidden as much as they just need to be found. It's no different than the autism journey. A child is sick or in some kind of need. This means it is more than likely up to the parent to lead the way of finding the answers, and not necessarily just pharmaceutical remedies.

---

[1]   Courtesy of the Thinking Moms' Revolution, http://thinkingmomsrevolution.
com/.

One of my daughter's friends lost her father to cancer. A day before he passed, I was asked by her mother to have her come to our house after school since the girl has a blood disorder that requires great care. While I have not been schooled in this disorder, I knew enough about nutrition to fully understand how her immune system was being impacted; not just by the disorder, but her own eating habits which were compromising her health. When this young girl started coming to our house (every weekday for six months), it was my task to monitor how she was coping and inform her mother if anything was needed. She would often not eat during the day, except for a bag of chips, and then come to my home with low energy. Slowly, I got her to see how she was not just affecting her health today but probably long term. So I began to show her how to make a quick snack that had good nutrition and to drink plenty of water. In spite of the difficulty she experienced with losing her father, she actually began to put on weight and grow (something she needed to do).

The theme in this is that all disease, disorders, and other health issues usually have a direct correlation to something that is probably fixable with the right interventions. This is not just wishful thinking. There are a throng of parents, physicians, and therapists who believe the same thing. We are just beginning to fully appreciate where a new outlook on medical practices will take us. And none too soon. We are on the precipice of true knowledge, especially with how to heal our children.

Chapter Four

You Are the Savvy Expert on Your Child, and Other Time-Worn Truths

"Mrs. Romaniec, what is your medical background?" asked the head of immunology at a leading children's hospital. As he flipped through the chronological notes that detailed my son's extensive medical history, he had asked the question with a glint of amazement.

"Doctor, I am the mother of a child with autism. The lab lives in my house," was the reply that seemed to roll off my tongue like there should have been a degree framed and displayed in my kitchen at home. It was true. I was a savvy expert on any and all things that pertained to my son.

As mentioned earlier, I coined the phrase "You are the CEO, your child is the company" as the analogy of who parents need to be when representing anything and everything that pertained to their child. Call it CEO, president, captain, head coach, lead advocate, medical director . . . you name it. All acronyms and analogies apply as long as it pertains to the idea that a parent leads and is fully in charge of their child's health, education, and well-being.

While all of that may seem like a given mindset, the reality is when parents of children with autism are faced with the diagnosis there is a very real sense that they are supposed to defer to any and all other authority figures. This means that in the eyes of the capitulating parent, the doctors know more, the therapists know more, the schools know more. Until the parent realizes how crucial it is to change that mindset will they begin to move away from the idea that they have no control over their child's situation. They definitely have more expertise and intuition on what is going on with their child. They just need to be reminded why this is, even more so when their child is diagnosed with autism.

While elements of this thought process were discussed in the previous chapter, I have separated out this section to highlight because of how often parents fall into the trap that, because someone has a degree or a title after their name, somehow their opinion as parents no longer counts. This chapter segues from the previous two chapters to discuss ways to have conversations with the experts and authorities involved with the child's care. We tend to relinquish our intellect, gut instincts, and wherewithal when dealing with the imposing authority of those with medical/professional credentials.

It is also my hope that physicians read this chapter to realize that parents are savvy these days. Rather than ridicule our research efforts, physicians and therapists should be joining in the effort and encouraging diverse opinions so that true understanding of how to help children and family impacted by autism is realized.

Why Professionals Are Burning Out and How That Impacts Your Child

Many of my friends are in the medical profession. They are dedicated, hard-working, and incredibly caring. They are also tired and frustrated. All of them. It comes with the territory that medical professionals today are commodities in the grand scheme of ensuring the profit margins are maintained or widened. Their caseloads are increased and their support system is decreased. They are held to a standard that is almost impossible to achieve. They are expected to spend fifteen minutes with a patient, diagnose accurately, order tests, perform procedures, submit copious paperwork, answer to case workers and hospital administrators, and be sure to be all things to everyone who needs their attention. Many are able to juggle what is expected of them, but many fall way short and end up taking it out on the very people they are supposed to serve—their patients.

A 2014 *Wall Street Journal* article[1] went into detail on how doctor burnout is now an epidemic. The writer explained that, because of the time constraints and fiscal challenges of the healthcare environment, doctors were walking away from their profession in droves. Those that remained were not doing what they had hoped when they graduated medical school. They saw everything they opposed in the healthcare system become the norm, meaning they were losing the personal human moments that only come with a trusted doctor-patient relationship.

They are becoming more challenged by their patients who have a vested interest in finding the answers for themselves or their loved one, while the doctors often do not have the time to do the same level of research unless it is their field of specialty. This, in turn, has led many in the medical profession to criticize patients who do Google research and chastise them for seeking answers outside of the doctor's knowledge base. Now throw in autism and you can see why many doctors have become frustrated with savvy autism parents. We research, we ask questions, and we are not afraid to disagree or seek a different approach to treating autism. For doctors who are in the realm of wanting something "cured," they are at a loss on what to do for the child with autism because their profession tells them there is no cure, which leaves the doctor scrambling to find something to alleviate the symptoms but not get to the bottom of what is causing the symptoms.

And that is the conundrum that parents face when they begin to seek the answers for their child. They feel they are supposed to go to one type of doctor or another, when the medical model is not yet established to have the answers.

As a pediatric neurologist explained, if you have a child with seizures, you take them to a neurologist. However, if your child also presents with gastrointestinal issues then you take them to the gastroenterologist. And if your child has an immune system issue, you go to the immunologist. But the thing with autism is that they are all related. One begets the other. Gut issues lead to neurological and immune system issues, which leads back to gut issues.

---

1   Sandeep Jauhar, "Why Doctors Are Sick of Their Profession," The Wall Street Journal, August 29, 2014, http://www.wsj.com/articles/the-u-s-s-ailing-medical-system-a-doctors-perspective-1409325361.

Then you have a myriad of behaviors and comorbidities that must be addressed by other experts like behavior specialists, physical therapists, speech pathologists, and occupational therapists.

So we become the expert in all modalities of treating our child because we have to. Now toss in the burnt-out physician or therapist who has to answer to higher-ups, all while juggling an unreasonable schedule. An autism parent comes in the door with an armload of information and concerns they want addressed, but the burnt-out professional puts up the stop sign. Mostly, it is out of their purview, or they relegate the conversation to what they always do within the traditional model.

When Daniel was around two years old, he was in anguish with his gastrointestinal pain. We finally secured an appointment with a well-known gastroenterologist and she agreed to do an endoscopy on him. When I pushed to have a colonoscopy done on him as well to figure out the reason for his chronic diarrhea (now going on fifteen months of non-stop diarrhea) she refused, telling me that he did not have blood in his stool so she would not do a colonoscopy. This was frustrating because I knew the problems and answers would be found in his gut but she refused due to some medical protocol that would leave us looking for answers somewhere else.

The endoscopy showed significant erosion of the esophagus, stomach, and upper intestine, for which she prescribed medication. She could not define what had caused the erosion, but I found out later when I was doing Google research (insert irony), which led to a published medical study that said too much soy can lead to this kind of erosion. Considering soy was a staple in Daniel's diet, it was evident we now needed to remove it since it was possibly causing his gut issues. Within a day of removing the soy all of his late-night writhing and screams of pain stopped. Granted, we had also started the medication, so it was hard to tell right away if it was working until we stopped the medication and the pain did not return.

I later found out that this same doctor had embraced a change in medical protocol and began to do colonoscopies on children with autism, even when they did not present with blood in the stool. I had also heard that she was working side by side with one of the top pediatric gastroenterologists in the country to learn more about the kids with autism, probably because they were becoming her largest clientele. While she presented to me as disengaged and disinterested, I was glad to hear she had turned around the apathy to help the next generation of children.

Even doctors who specialize in autism, also known as MAPS or DAN doctors, burnout or become apathetic. I spoke with one of these doctors to let him know he needed to get to the conferences and begin educating himself on the latest treatments because the parents of his patients were outpacing him in knowledge. He was way behind, I told him.

Other professionals who work with our children also get burnt out and leave their professions. This is especially true of behavior therapists, also known as Applied Behavior Analysis (ABA) providers. As wide-eyed, full of purpose college students, they gravitate to working with children with autism because they sincerely want to make a difference. And they do. But what they don't count on is that their caseloads will be more than they can handle; they will be expected to travel, and completing paperwork will be their second job. I know this because I receive emails from college students who are looking to work in the profession, and they are always encouraged by me to pursue their profession because of the tremendous need for therapists. But I also wonder how long they will actually last.

This can be a lucrative profession for some, earning upwards of fifty dollars an hour. The average therapist fresh out of college will earn half that amount. Our children are not the easiest to deal with at times, but the right therapist can make a difference. It's a matter of finding—and keeping—the right one.

Speech pathologists at school are another commodity ripe for burnout. One of my friends is a speech pathologist and she has absolutely no time to do a proper job, in her eyes. She has a full caseload at a school district, but as more kids are diagnosed they simply just add them to her workload rather than hire a new pathologist. Over time, she knew she was not servicing her students well, and certainly not to their IEPs, because her caseload was too full. The only thing that stopped it was a parent sued the school district and brought them to Due Process which mediates IEP violations and services not offered or followed. The attorney spent a lot of time with my friend and asked her to detail her day. She admitted in court that she was given a caseload that required students be seen in thirty minute sessions, but in reality she provided them fifteen minutes because she had too many students. And this did not include the time away to attend meetings or fill in paperwork, which she often did outside the regular school day. Needless to say, the district lost the case and was significantly reprimanded for allowing the situation to occur, and for so many children to not be properly served.

In another district, instead of providing adequate services with trained professionals they opted to bring in regular substitute teachers to do the therapy, at eight dollars an hour. The parents found out about it and notified the principals and superintendents that their child needed to have their services made up by qualified therapists. The school district knew they were caught doing something illegal and indeed re-did the therapy sessions for the students involved. It was the expert parents that held them accountable, citing word and verse of state law on the matter.

If a Professional Implies "My Way or the Highway," Choose the Highway

Intimidation by medical professionals is rampant within the autism community. How often have I heard from other parents about the physician, therapist, or others who gave them ultimatums or risk being asked to leave the practice. I have even experienced this myself. This is especially true with the sacred cow of vaccine protocol. Pediatricians are quick to say that unless the parent complies with the full American Academy of Pediatrics (AAP) recommended vaccine schedule, then the pediatrician will dismiss the family from the practice. End of story to them, and they think that if enough pediatricians join ranks (about a third now do this) that all parents will be forced to comply or not have anyone to go to.

But here's the quick question I ask every parent who believes this is a dilemma: Why do you as a parent choose to stay? You don't think you will find another physician who will actually listen to you? Since when does your opinion count less than the "expert" on what is right for your child? It isn't that they have a preference for the choice that you make but rather that they insist on it by delivering an ultimatum. As I was writing this chapter, legislation was making its way in numerous states to remove religious exemption as a reason for a vaccine waiver. Where the measures were defeated, parents had actively protested against the intrusive nature of the bills in question; especially since it meant that they did not have full say in medical decisions for their children.

This section, then, deals with the traits of audacity and assertiveness. Parents must learn to recognize bullies with fancy credentials after their names, learn not be intimidated, and instead make decisions that are right for their child and family.

Before we moved to Massachusetts from California, and before Daniel lost his diagnosis, I began to look for an ABA provider in the new area. One was apparently a well-known ABA school, so I was excited to speak to them about our move and taking Daniel on as a client. The woman on the other end of the phone could not have been drier when she explained how I would have to sign an affidavit that we would not pursue diet or biomedical treatments while receiving ABA services from the school. Come again?

"Um, my son is gluten and dairy free and needs to continue to be," I said. She replied that unless I brought in a note from a doctor stipulating the need to be gluten and dairy free then they would theoretically feed him the food he was not supposed to eat. They used food as rewards, so the crappy GMO, artificial everything snacks would be fed to my son.

"So what you are saying is that my opinion as the parent has no bearing?" I continued in a heightened state of voice to say, "You think you know more about my son than I do?!" The worst part about that place was how many parents actually *signed* an affidavit saying they would not follow their own parental instincts and implement a diet or pursue biomedical treatments. They worded it differently, but that is exactly what a parent was signing. Obviously, I chose the highway rather than this place.

I was at the playground with my two children when I noticed a little boy who was by himself and not engaging with the other children. I asked my children to go make friends with him and play if he wanted to. The mother of the boy came over to thank me and explained that he had autism. I introduced myself and pointed out that my son was recovered from autism, which intrigued her because the whole idea of recovery was still not talked about. I told her our story of diet and the use of IVIG to repair his damaged immune system. She nodded her head, saying that she had wanted to investigate IVIG for her son too, because he presented with so many immune issues. He seemed like he should at least be tested for it. But she was given an ultimatum by a developmental pediatrician that if the mother pursued anything outside of behavior therapy then the doctor would no longer see the patient. So the mother stopped pursing further research and testing. She gave me a shrug as if to say "What was I to do?" or "Oh well." My response was, "And you bought that?! That's too bad." I went on to say that no doctor should ever have that much control over the decisions we make for our children. But, of course, this was falling on deaf ears and our conversation quickly ended.

When my youngest was born in 2006, we had ultrasound evidence that he was coming in with a couple of birth defects, including hypospadias (a penis defect) and a kidney dysfunction known as hydronephrosis (fluid in the kidney). We had already decided that due to Daniel's vaccine reaction, we were not going to have our newborn vaccinated—at all. The laws in Massachusetts are pretty liberal when it comes to parental birth orders at hospitals, so we stipulated no vitamin K, no hepatitis B, and nothing in his eyes. The OB physician had no problem with the request and ordered a series of tests to be done on our newborn after he was born. We also had a pediatric urologist lined up to order necessary testing on his kidneys once he was born.

A C-section was planned because we had significant complications with the birth of my older two children, and at almost forty-four, I knew the risk of a difficult labor would make it tougher on the baby and me. David was born via C-section at 6:29 p.m. When I was in recovery, I began to have a bad reaction to the morphine and was shaking all over. Simultaneous to this reaction a call came in to the nurse's station in the recovery room from the on-call pediatrician who wanted to question my decision to not give our son vitamin K, explaining the complications of potential brain bleed. She added later that she "accepted" the decision to not do the hepatitis B vaccine since the delivery was C-section. Believe me, I had a lot of things I wanted to say during this part of the conversation. I told her the vitamin K contained aluminum and since our family has a predisposition to having a problem excreting heavy metals we were forgoing vitamin K.

She was annoyed, insisting there was no aluminum in vitamin K and suggesting that the benefits far outweighed the risks of aluminum. I replied, "Doctor, you have no idea about our family's risk levels." We continued our back and forth conversation for forty-five minutes, with me shaking the whole time from the morphine reaction, before the nurses took the phone away and pointedly told the doctor that she needed to abide by the parent's wishes.

The doctor had also insisted that the hospital pharmacist had said there was no aluminum in vitamin K and had no purpose for being there any way. I asked the doctor to please send the vitamin K package insert to the room once I was assigned. She explained that she had six hours to get the vitamin K in him or risk brain bleed (total panic on her part, so this must have been drilled into her during medical school). Although she did admit that vitamin K did not become routinely used in newborns in the US until the early 1970s, and she and I did not receive vitamin K at birth.

By 10:30 p.m., I was finally recovered enough to go to my own room. The vitamin K package insert arrived almost right away and in it was this section:

> WARNING: This product contains aluminum that may be toxic. Aluminum may reach toxic levels with prolonged parenteral administration if kidney function is impaired. Premature neonates are particularly at risk because their kidneys are immature, and they required large amounts of calcium and phosphate solutions, which contain aluminum.
>
> Research indicates that patients with impaired kidney function, including premature neonates, who receive parenteral levels of aluminum at greater than 4 to 5 mcg/kg/day accumulate aluminum at levels associated with central nervous system and bone toxicity. Tissue loading may occur at even lower rates of administration.

Oh boy. Clear as day, and not one of them took the time to read it. How many other children with kidney dysfunction were potentially harmed? Maybe none, but we will never know because doctors and pharmacists are unaware that this is something to consider before administering it to a newborn with kidney dysfunction.

At midnight, I received the last attempt at persuasion by the pediatrician and I read off the warning in the insert to her. She was undeterred and again said the benefits outweighed the risks. I then told her no again and she said that as a result of the decision she planned to write up an affidavit against me and put it in my son's medical records. Incensed at the intimidation tactic that was also meant to protect herself, I fired off that I would be writing up my own affidavit which I wanted typed, stapled to the package insert, and put into the files too. And this is exactly what happened.

The nurses I met in the labor and delivery area were all wonderful and gave me reassurance on the decision, with a show of admiration, evident by how many nurses came to talk to me on the topic of vaccines over the next few days. When David was brought downstairs for his first scan on his kidney function, I discovered that even the nurses there had heard of my showdown with the pediatrician. They also felt that there were too many vaccines being given, and too early. I don't think it was so much the vaccine debate that generated the interest as it was that I stood my ground against what was an obvious bully tactic, something they must have seen with other parents, and I was the one who would not back down.

A month later, the US Health and Human Services Department issued a warning to all hospitals about vitamin K containing aluminum and stated that it should be used with caution with newborns who presented with kidney dysfunction. It was bittersweet vindication, only because I knew hospitals would continue to ignore the warning.

There are a number of parents I know who have become so knowledgeable on all things pertaining to their child's needs that they run circles around physicians, therapists, and school district personnel. But there are many more who have taken a back seat to what their role is supposed to be. They arrive at doctors or therapy appointments unprepared to participate in a real discussion because they have not done any research or lined up their questions. They fully expect the professional to arrive at conclusions and dish out the answers for them, which rankles me because it means the parents have chosen the path of least resistance. This does not mean that the professional's ideas are not sound and fully in order with what is necessary for the child, but that the parent needs to engage in the process.

I have also heard from enough parents who fear what their spouse would say if they did any of their own research and not just blindly follow a recommendation. There would potentially be a disagreement between the couple based on the idea that a parent is taking a proactive role in opposition to just deferring to traditional medical opinions.

Some parents arrive ready to record or videotape appointments so as not to miss a single bit of the appointment. In contrast, a woman I mentored was tremendously disappointed in the physician I recommended because the doctor didn't have any real information except the lab results. The more I peppered her with questions the more I realized she had expected the doctor to just roll out the red carpet that would lead to full recovery for her child. There are some physicians who have that ability to create a road map that may lead to recovery, but most need more input from the parents and more time to discern long-term options.

I understood her expectations, especially when we tend to spend a lot of money for these appointments, testing, and treatments. But I also realized she had arrived ill-prepared to ask questions, speak to new concerns, and adjust priorities, and she didn't press the doctor on how to follow up based on the results of the labs. Yes, it is natural to assume the doctor should have known, but the mother needed to shift her perspective on her role in the matter. She needed to be a partner in the process of finding answers for her child.

When Daniel needed sound therapy to address his auditory processing delay, we took him to a facility that was sixty-eight miles away. We came prepared to ask questions but also knew how this particular therapy differed from others that were similar. The other forms of treatment were not as expensive or as intense as this one, but by the time we ended our consultation session, both Rich and I were convinced this was the treatment he needed. It turned out to be a decision that had lasting benefits.

A friend of mine was certain her son had a health issue with potential genetic origins, and pushed the physicians to test him and her other child for the MTHFR gene, which is highly implicated in families that have a child with autism. As it turned out, her son had a total deletion of the gene which is part of the cycle that helps our bodies detoxify (methylate), meaning his body did not have the ability to detox his environmental toxins, on top of complications with his immune system and mental health disorders.

One of Daniel's doctors suggested that he be tested for MTHFR as well. When the lab result came back positive, I immediately scoured the internet for information and then scheduled an appointment to have me and our other two children tested. I discovered that we are all positive for a variation of this gene, and this discovery led to us changing the supplements we took. We then focused on long-term changes that we needed to make in the wake of knowing our genetic predisposition to certain disorders.

What is important is to define who we are as parents in this progression. If you take a secondary role, you may end up with secondary results.

When the Ego Walks In the Door First

Over the years, we have had to seek out some top-notch doctors, as far as their reputations were concerned. Many of them were esteemed in their profession, by their colleagues as well as the parents in the autism community. What I found was that while some deserved these noteworthy reputations, others clearly were more impressed with themselves and just trusted you would be too. I mean, why else seek an appointment with the doctor if you didn't realize how important they were? Ahem.

One of the first appointments with this kind of doctor was the head of the pediatric orthopedics department of a university hospital. Daniel was eight months old, and this specialist was to determine if he was going to eventually need surgery for his bilateral club foot. The recent X-rays of his feet were put up by the medical student who did the initial intake, and then we waited another twenty minutes or so for the doctor. His entrance was as though the King of Siam had arrived with a bevy of medical students surrounding him, his entire demeanor signifying he knew he was important. The medical students crammed into the small room, taking notes on the advice he was giving us.

First, he examined Daniel's feet, made some comment and then went to look at the X-ray. "Ah, that's good," he said. "Right on target. He is at an eighty-five degree angle."

I looked at the X-ray and immediately saw the problem. "Uh, doctor." I grabbed the X-ray, flipped it around and right side up and said, "That's a twenty-eight degree angle."

Flustered, the doctor backtracked and said, "Oh yes, that's right." Then he carried on like nothing had happened. But I looked around at the medical students and wondered how much of this exchange they had noted, as in their hero worship might have just been deflated a bit.

When we later had to consult yet another orthopedic specialist, he kept us waiting for three hours. I wondered what would happen if we had showed up for the appointment late by three hours. There was no advance phone call that the doctor was running that far behind, nor was there a way for us to leave and come back when the doctor was close to being able to see us. That's just how it was at this place. The doctor was chronically behind, and patients were made to linger in the waiting room with no way of knowing when the doctor would be available. Many left without being seen. We would have too if not for the fact we had waited months to see this specialist.

When we met him, we understood why he ran behind. He liked to talk about himself. He offered no advice except to suggest we wait until Daniel had reached puberty to determine if he would need surgery on his heel cords (waiting was good enough for us), but otherwise it was a useless appointment. We were baffled on how this doctor had earned such a stellar reputation when our experience was anything but positive.

That said, there are many physicians that you may not have heard much about but who are perfect for your child and your family. You develop a relationship with them and they listen to your needs. Well, that's the hope. They are out there and they are worth finding.

You Are the CEO, and Your Child Is the Company

Quite a while ago, I wrote magazine article called "Closing the IEP Deal," which outlined the idea that IEP meetings are like business negotiations, only with the child's needs coming out on top. The article struck a chord; I later found it on other special needs websites and even attorney websites as a reference for their clients.

I touched on elements of this in chapter 2, but a portion of this needs to be expanded upon in the context of how you conduct yourself professionally with the school district, respond to any bullying tactics, and ensure you are always, always looking out for your child's well-being. The strategies that I intuitively employed were plain old business strategies that I dusted off from my corporate days.

My personal journey as CEO of my child's care began when my husband and I were getting ready to head into Daniel's first IEP meeting. I had previously met with the district as part of the transition period before Daniel turned three, which was when the school district would take over services from the early intervention agency. While I was on top all of Daniel's medical and therapy appointments, the school stuff was completely out of my realm of understanding. But as luck would have it, I attended a meeting with a special needs attorney who spoke about all of the things parents do wrong in the IEP process. And I was the total poster child for everything he was talking about.

The attorney paced the room in a droll sort of way and laid out how parents arrive at IEP meetings completely unprepared (check), believed the school district will just do the right thing (double check), did not write letters to express concern or confirm a conversation (oh Lord, I had not written any at that stage), tried to make friends with the school district personnel (you mean we're not supposed to?), and forget that their job was to advocate for their child. By the end of his presentation, I was a changed woman. Holy cow! This was Business 101 all over again, and I had three weeks to get good at this process for the sake of my son.

That day, I bought a book called *The Complete IEP Guide* by Lawrence Siegel, a special education attorney. The book was filled with templates for letters to write and details on special education law. I got it and immediately understood what I needed to do. The poor school district personnel had little idea what they were in for because by Monday morning I began the letter writing campaign and getting engaged with the whole process. I sent or dropped off a total of nine letters in two weeks outlining concerns, making requests, and in all other ways letting them know that this mom was going to be involved with the IEP. I wasn't trying to be a nuisance, but I invariably became one.

The school district made it plain that they were aiming to put Daniel in a special day class for children with autism. Knowing that Daniel had the ability to emulate typical behavior, there was no way he was not going to be with peers in a regular preschool classroom setting. So they had me look at the Head Start program on one of their school campuses, and that was even worse. There were twenty-four students, two teachers, and a classroom aide, mixed with a lot of chaos. The noise level alone was more than I could handle, so there was no way my son with autism would be able to handle it. No, the only option was going to be private preschool with a shadow aide that the district would then pay for.

The school district psychologist was sent to our house to evaluate Daniel, and I innately knew he was trying to mitigate Daniel's abilities in order to say that the special day class was the only appropriate setting for him. This irked me, and the psychologist's behavior in our home was so bizarre that I notified the early intervention agency of his interaction. They called the school district to suggest he be removed from Daniel's case, which the district did. This particular psychologist, however, had a slippery reputation amongst those in the local special needs parent community. "Beware of his tricks," I was warned.

I was unsure what this meant until, just before departing, the psychologist had given me a questionnaire to fill out in order to complete Daniel's initial evaluations. Since the psychologist clearly had a biased slant against Daniel, I went through the questionnaire thoroughly and realized that he had given me a test for a child that was at least five years older. The data would have been skewed to suggest that Daniel was more impaired and therefore belonged in the special day class. Now I was on high alert. In my mind, this was purposeful subterfuge, and they were dealing with the wrong mother.

The gloves were off. I was now a woman on a mission, and that mission was urgent! I had to be the captain of my son's IEP team and, as such, be in charge of how this first meeting was going to be run. I learned all I could about some of the people at the school who would be involved in the IEP process. I then turned my attention to developing clear objectives in my mind as to what services we wanted for our son. This was a high-profile business project all over again. Only, now I was the CEO and my son was the company.

With well-defined program goals in mind, the letter writing continued. I sent a letter objecting to anyone attending the meeting without first meeting my son, as well as objecting to anyone attending who did not have a specific purpose at the IEP meeting. I had learned early on in the business world that one common negotiation tactic to show dominance was to stack the room with "your guys" so that your people outnumbered theirs, even if half of them were silent during the meeting. Other parents had mentioned that several specialists from the district were often asked to participate in IEP meetings for kids they had not even met, just to provide an indication of support for the watered down proposal from the school district. Well, this was at least the practice when we first began to have IEP meetings. Over the years, the number of people in the room waned because they were flat out too busy with their caseloads just to be another voice in the room. At the time, however, I was feeling a sense of déjà vu, and the old business meeting tendencies kicked in.

In my letter, I stated that if they had not evaluated him then they would not serve a purpose (yes, I was a tad arrogant and using my audacious, assertiveness attributes). This caught the district by surprise since the district special education administrator was slated to be in the room, even though she was not scheduled to evaluate or meet either me or Daniel in advance of the meeting. So I called her to ask her to come to our home. I was polite and told her my concerns with her not meeting my son in advance was that she would not get the picture of why I was advocating for a preschool setting where he would be able to emulate typical peers. Amazingly, she came and was very cordial, spending maybe fifteen minutes at the house. Truthfully, I also knew she was sizing me up just as much as Daniel.

By the time the first IEP meeting happened, I was on edge. This was the biggest "business" meeting I had ever participated in, and the stakes were higher: my son's well-being. But when I arrived at the meeting, there were fourteen school district people, my husband, our early intervention contact, and Daniel's physical therapist. There were tape recorders out since I had requested the meeting be recorded, and large post-it note style poster paper. The poster paper was not foreign to me since I had used it often in business meetings for strategy sessions. But the early intervention person looked at them with disbelief. I found out later it was because she had never seen a district go through this level of effort in an IEP meeting.

As the meeting got underway, there was a lot of give and take, which was carefully logged on the poster paper that eventually began to take over the room. At the end of three hours there were over a dozen large poster sheets filled in with every possible consideration to ensure Daniel's needs were met. But they were still trying to figure out a way to keep from moving him out of district.

"We *always* place the first year students in the special day class," the special education finally said.

"What you are suggesting," I replied, "is a one-size-fits-all program and my son is entitled to an *individual* education plan." She said no more the rest of the meeting, but it gave me pause as to how many parents are told this nonsense that the school district protocol overrode the child's needs. Sadly I would see this play out in the years to come with other children.

At the end of the meeting, the early intervention person took me aside and said, "I have never seen anything like that."

"What do you mean?" I responded. "The meeting? What was different about it?"

She said, "They made it high profile." Not understanding what she was saying, I asked what she thought caused it to become high profile. "You," she said with emphasis.

That's just it; I didn't know what I was doing so I did everything I thought I should. Again, I reflected back on my former profession and realized that I just incorporated those same instincts when it mattered most.

Still, it took four additional IEP meetings, where we went round and round on the outside placement and speech therapy. I finally got fed up with what I thought were games being played to stall the implementation of Daniel's IEP before the school year began. I called the special education director, the same one who had come to my home, and in a firm tone I said, "Look, Trudy*, I see the tactics you are doing to stall this process. So feel free to do whatever you have to do to make yourself look good to the higher-ups. Make it look like you took me to the mat, as long as you know that my son comes out with what he needs in the end."

She replied by acknowledging what she was facing in the district (behind the scenes politics). She asked me to give her until after her vacation the following week to come back with the plan in place. I told her that was fine as long as Daniel ended up with exactly what he needed (namely, what I asked for).

"You see, Trudy, I am the mom who will take you to Due Process and I am the mom who will win," I added. Okay, I probably would not say that now as readily as I did then because Due Process has become more difficult than it used to, and it is definitely harder in some states.

Two weeks later, a mediation meeting was called to finalize the IEP. The only problem was the mediator that needed to fly in from Sacramento got the time mixed up and did not arrive on time. So I mediated with just the school district personnel who tried to use the old analogy of "We are only required to give you a Chevy education plan, not a Cadillac." I hate that phrase because of how stupid it sounds and how often it is repeated.

"Look," I replied, "let's dog pile on my son now so that he doesn't need you one day. What is it going to take to get him to kindergarten on time? That is what we are aiming for." They said little else after that, and we ended up signing the agreement. It was exactly what I had asked for in the first IEP meeting, only this one had one-on-one speech therapy and they had to reimburse me for the outside speech evaluation.

During coffee klatch with my fellow autism friends, I told the story of our IEP meetings and something about it caught the ear of other parents outside the klatch, and the next thing I knew I was getting calls from total strangers asking if I would show them what to do for their child. It was odd since I felt I knew so little about IEPs. But eventually I did start advocating with other parents, or mentoring them on how to advocate since they needed to be the one to have a strong, long-term relationship with the school district.

When I began to mentor more, it seemed that mentoring provided a natural springboard to discuss diet, biomedical therapies, and then eventually get into the subject of their child's IEP or the school district. One mother I mentored was a first generation American of Asian descent who had a four-year-old daughter with severe autism, needing significant interventions. First, I gave the mother information on diet, and then as she was approaching the first IEP meeting she asked for input, which I gave her, including not signing the IEP at the first meeting.

The call I received later that week stunned me. The school district was going to provide four hours a week of services—for everything! That was speech, some ABA, and some OT, all in the span of four hours a week, which was completely unacceptable for any preschool age child on the spectrum, let alone one as severe as her daughter.

"You didn't sign that agreement did you," I implored.

"Yes, I did. I didn't know what else to do," she said in anguish.

That was when I knew the district had taken advantage of her as a first-generation American, knowing that, because of her cultural background, she was likely to defer to authority figures. I have witnessed districts throughout the country later do this with Hispanic and low-income families. They had sized her up as the parent who would not fight them. And in a way they were right. Only, they were about to be shown how very wrong they were in this situation.

"You renege," I screamed into the phone. "Renege, renege, renege! And when you do that, I am putting you in touch with an attorney I know. He will make sure this is fixed."

By this stage I was pacing the floor. They were trying to screw a kid! And they thought they would get away with it. I knew she would be in good hands with the attorney I recommended because he was the one I heard speak that fateful day at a meeting a couple of years earlier.

Six weeks later, I heard from this mother to tell me the outcome of the meeting with the attorney. The attorney was so incensed at the flagrant violation of this child's rights that he immediately took the case, sent the mother to have the child evaluated by a number of top-notch experts in their field in a matter of days. To give you an idea of how unheard of this is, it takes months to get appointments with most of these experts. But when a high-powered attorney who sends a lot of clients your way calls and says drop everything I have an urgent case, they drop what they are doing and make room for the client. That's what happened in this case.

Within six weeks, they were in Due Process with the attorney and the school district. Six weeks! That is incredibly soon after a case is received that it ends up in Due Process. This reflects how badly this school district botched this one. The attorney for the school district hung his head and leaned over to the special education director and said, "How did you let this happen?" There was never a need to call witnesses or present their case because the district's attorney recommended full acceptance of the findings and whatever services were asked for the child. This included an $80,000 a year out-of-district school placement, busing, outside therapies, and, of course, legal bills reimbursed. The mother was beyond thrilled. Her daughter was in a comprehensive program, finally receiving services she needed. And the mother felt vindicated.

My rapport with a variety of therapists and others connected with this girl encouraged them to ask for my input on how to get the mother to trust them again. They knew the district blew it, but those on the ground working with her had their hearts in the right place and wanted to help her. While I felt for them, I understood where the mother was coming from. So I suggested they begin by offering her something she hadn't asked for, listening to her concerns, and then only slowly begin building that bridge again. I moved shortly after so I don't know the final outcome, but I hope that this is what happened and that the girl went on to succeed. The district no doubt learned a lesson, and I was made aware of how districts size up parents in order to determine how likely they will be to fight back.

Tips for Dealing with Any and All Professionals Working with Your Child

1. **Arrive prepared** to ask questions and offer input. Whether you are speaking with your child's doctor, a therapist, or a school district administrator, always arrive prepared to have a full conversation with the end goal of getting your child to the next level of well-being and achievement.

2. **Get educated** on what is available, whether it is a medical treatment, therapy, or educational model. How do you know what to ask for if you don't know what is available? I found the best resources to be other parents that I met online or through a variety of networks. What worked for one child might be worth looking into for mine, and so on.

3. **Put it in writing**. Most professionals consider a well-written letter that is respectful, concise, and well thought out as a measurement of the responsiveness of the parent. If you are willing to write a letter, then you are willing to engage in the process of helping your child. I often have heard from parents who find writing a letter difficult and would rather pay attorneys and advocates to do their bidding. But letter writing is the biggest tool a parent has to be their child's best advocate. It is essential.

4. **Act in a business-like manner**. If a therapist, physician, or other expert was gauging how they helped my son

by what they thought of me, then I was going to be the one to act in a professional manner. I dressed for the occasion, meaning more than my ratty house-cleaning clothes, and affirmed my business manners (well, as long as they did). I also made for sure that I did not try to be their friends while they were working for my son. It was a dividing line I knew would put them in an awkward position, so I never breached that trust and maintained a respectful decorum that was not overly personal. Chances are that twenty years from now they will not be in your child's life. But you will.

5. **Be organized.** The paperwork mountain will overwhelm you, which is why it is necessary to keep all of your medical and educational records on hand. This part is discussed in detail in chapter 8, but just know that organization can make or break your long-term effort and cause unnecessary stress if it is lacking.

6. **Be scrupulous with your word.** If you are given information in confidence from a professional, keep it that way. Do not betray their trust. Use the information to help your child or to make decisions. Do not use it as fodder for gossip. This goes a long way in ensuring they trust you with more information when the time comes.

7. **Listen to their input.** We need to have a respectful give-and-take with those who are connected with helping our child. Ideally, it is a respectful conversation exchanging ideas and information. Don't be afraid to ask for their input, even if they don't offer it initially. It shows you value their opinion too.

8. **Know when to end a relationship that is not working.** If a professional of any sort fails to provide answers, or your child is no longer making progress through their interventions, then it is time to find someone else. This is another reason to keep a respectful distance without complicating your rapport. You need to stay focused on your child's needs, not the feelings of the professional you pay.

Why Bother?

I have mentored many families over the years, and the biggest challenge for them is understanding that how they conduct themselves may affect how treatment and services are provided for their children. This is *not* to say that professionals ever take out their angst on a child rather than a parent. But I can tell you that you are being sized up at all times, whether others will tell you that or not. This is about the attributes we acquire and the mantras we adopt too.

When a father of triplets called me for advice on the upcoming IEPs (yes, three different meetings), he wondered what his approach with the team should be.

"Should I come in guns blazing?" he asked.

"No, you come in like you are the CEO representing your company with professionalism and certainty. You know what is needed for your company(ies) to grow and succeed. That is what you do. Always."

Chapter Five

I Want to Be a Girlfriend Again! Overcoming Grief's Impact on the Marriage

What is it about married life that drives the sexy right out of us? While sex still happens, the bachelorette party lingerie sits in the bottom drawer (as my married friends had warned me it would before the first anniversary). There were days when I yearned to be treated like a sexy girlfriend again. And if the short skirts still fit, I'd wear them too.

Within a few short years of marriage, my reality was far removed from sexy girlfriend thoughts. It's amazing that at one point all of that non-important, truly stupid stuff mattered. That is, until Daniel was diagnosed with autism at the age of eighteen months. Our daughter Theresa was just fourteen months old when Daniel was born, leaving me in a permanent state of exhaustion over the next few years from caring for two young children. The diagnosis itself seemed almost a relief, an answer at least, to the mind-numbing behaviors and health issues our son was going through almost from the moment he was born. Nothing in our marriage vows prepared us for this kind of "for better or for *worse*" of watching our son writhe on the ground from stomach pain, and us feeling powerless to help him. With autism, thoughts of a normal life, let alone girlfriend treatment, were instantly replaced by survival instincts.

With the diagnosis, Rich and I knew we were in an uphill battle for our son's future, with the side effect of not knowing

how all of this would impact our family. The ensuing grief began
to show up in our marriage, subtly at first, and then more overtly
as the stress and grief began to compound. Respectful conversations were practically gone as we squared off into two separate
emotional camps over the next year, with each of us certain that
we were alone in our personal battle. We were going through the
kind of grief similar to what comes with death or significant loss,
and neither one of us understood how to come to grips with it
all. Rich, for his part, still believed that the answers to Daniel's
well-being would be found solely in traditional medicine, and I
began to feel frustrated with the obvious. It wouldn't. More was
needed to help Daniel, and now I had to convince Rich too.

Conversations between Rich and me became borderline
nasty. We were either in battle mode or cautiously trying to find
peaceful ground. The no-man's-land was Daniel's escalating
health problems, including his incessant crying, chronic diarrhea
that had lingered since his first birthday, and stomach pains that
led to middle-of-the-night trips to the emergency room. At some
point, defining our individual roles became almost instinctual. I
became the designated researcher, therapist seeker, nutrition-
ist, and in all other ways an advocate for our son. Rich became
the champion of finding the ways to pay for whatever Daniel
needed. We were on autopilot. It felt better to just be doing
something as opposed to allowing the despair to take over, even
though there were days when it buried us, especially the days
when Daniel spent the day screaming, head-banging the floor,
or biting and pinching his sister.

Rich's late work schedule meant that tough conversations
didn't take place until ten o'clock at night, leading nowhere and
only adding to my anxiety and increasing his frustration levels.
In turn, I would spend long hours researching on the desktop
computer in our room, clacking at the keyboard well past midnight. Rich would sigh in exasperation and roll over with a pillow
over his head, letting me know that I was keeping him awake.

Morning routines after a sleep-deprived night often left me
in a blur of activity that "had to be done," or my job as mother
and caretaker would be a failure. Sexy girlfriend thoughts were
completely gone, as were all other thoughts that existed in a normal life, replaced by the narcotic of guilt just to get me through

the day. Guilt was what motivated me to keep up with the pace of handling the kids, the house, and all things autism . . . oh, and stifle my growing resentment in order to keep the peace at home.

A degree of indifference began to creep into our marriage. Sometimes, I begged and cajoled, and even manipulated, to have an evening out where autism was not the main topic of conversation. I longed to get dressed up with makeup and heels and head out, maybe even pull over just to make out (okay, I had wild long-ago fantasies brewing). Truly, I craved something "normal" to buffer the insanity of our lives, even if only a civil conversation in a parked car—once I got past the mental anguish and exhaustion.

But after a while, I gave up asking and just figured that *my* priority had to shift back to "more important" things, like the kids and our pending move to Massachusetts. Sex still happened and helped to keep us emotionally connected, but I wanted the predictable routine to be broken, maybe because it all seemed like a chummy co-existence. Couples who do not have a child with autism experience the same rut in their marriage. It's just that ours had a rut with no end in sight because *we were not important any more*, in our own eyes.

In my mentoring, I witnessed this same pattern of marital downward spiral take place in virtually every couple, some with more dire consequences, like the complete breakdown of their marriage and family. Worse was the eighty percent divorce rate discussed in autism circles as though it was a purple heart: not desired, but accepted. In mentoring, I would mention how sex was an important communication tool for couples who are in crisis because I saw its value in our own marriage. But what happens when the conversation is the same and little effort is made to change? What happens when lingering anger continues and sex stops all together, especially when we are dealing with the stress from a child who is ill? Eventually, the marital issues will come front and center for attention, some quicker than others. The trick is to bring the marriage needs to the forefront before a third party is needed to mediate: marriage counselor or divorce attorney.

Daniel lost his official diagnosis to autism by the age of four, and no two people could have been happier than me and Rich.

We knew that we still had a ways to go before he would be completely healed, but we also knew that the hard work and sacrifice had paid off with our son's return to health. On occasion, the thoughts of being a "girlfriend" again would resurface. Would we ever reclaim who we used to be? Did we even remember?

By the time we had our third child, David, we once again shifted into high gear to care for the needs of our son who would need his first of three surgeries by six months of age. Even after the move, and after both of our sons were on the road to recovery, Rich and I no longer discussed time together because the implication always was that we could not "afford" each other. Or more correctly put, our relationship was an unnecessary expense. I did, however, begin to wonder if money was the real reason for our aversion to connecting with each other, or just bad habits that had built up over time.

We were on course to become another statistic when I did the unthinkable. I brought our marriage to a screeching halt, or rather the current state of our marriage. With heartsickness welling in my throat, I shocked Rich when I told him that I intended to leave if our marriage did not change. We needed to reboot, or separate, simple as that. No longer could we afford to be on the back burner in priorities, and no longer could we afford to be disrespectful or condescending in our tones. We had to carve back into our psyches the idea that we once found each other sexy and fun. And we needed to become these people again to save our marriage.

Only by mending the rifts in our own marriage, through counseling and effort, did I understand the importance of what I had been preaching to other autism families. Angry and hurt, on the precipice of losing our marriage due to neglect, we needed to be reminded why we were a couple—and that we were still very much in love. "Do you remember what it was like when we were dating? I want us to be a boyfriend and girlfriend again." That became the slogan of our newly rebooted marriage; to remember that we were each other's boyfriend and girlfriend, even when we were mired in our daily duties.

In the middle of our marriage crisis, I read *The Seven Principles for Making Marriage Work: A Practical Guide from the Country's Foremost Relationship Expert*, by John M. Gottman and Nan

Silver, and found satisfaction in finding a shared philosophy. Specifically, they recommend that if you want a marriage to last you must be willing to end it (in its present form). I'm glad we did, because it saved us from ending our marriage permanently.

Let's Talk *Sex*!

Over the years of talking with couples—with women in particular—I have shared some chick-lit ideas of how we need to bring couples through the crisis of the grief cycle that hits after the autism diagnosis. In these conversations, there is a sudden flashback of who we used to be, before autism, back when we were sexy girlfriends and boyfriends. Sex works to bring a couple together. It's one of the reasons why we got married in the first place. It is not the only tool for greater communication and lasting changes, but it is a good bet that it is the one that gets our attention first.

At the 2005 Defeat Autism Now (DAN) conference in Boston, I was part of a parent panel. A woman in the packed audience stood up to ask how she could improve her marriage. I quickly took the microphone away from the doctor who was about to give an opinion on the issue, insisting I was the one to answer this question. I then offered advice on using sex as a communication tool. It seems that my strategy hit home because the audience's response included touchdown signs over the heads of the men, and women laughing at the absurdity of the obvious. Sex works! Now, if only we could remember how much fun we used to have doing it.

I told the story of Cindy, a friend and neighbor I was mentoring on diet and biomedical therapy for her son. She called to say she was furious at her husband for having fed her son gluten foods, which caused his autism behaviors to resurface the entire next day. Her son had been doing well on the gluten/casein-free diet, so this bad day seemed to her a frustrating setback. Cindy told me that when her husband got home she was planning to make his night as miserable as her day had been dealing with her son's out-of-control behaviors.

My girlfriend instinct kicked in and I told her to stop and rethink that idea.

"Instead of launching an attack on him, why not put the kids to bed early and give him a night he will not forget? And then, in the morning, gently mention to him how much you need his help to maintain your son on the diet. What do you think will get his attention more—nagging or great sex?"

Cindy was dumbfounded. Having sex with her husband was the farthest thing from her mind. She was mad! So I talked to her about needing her husband to not tune her out, and about getting his attention in a way he would remember. What was easy to realize from all of our conversations was that he was stuck between the stages of anger and denial, becoming angrier the more Cindy pushed him to accept all that she was doing for their son. He understood little that she told him except that his life, and that of his family's, was turned upside down by a roller-coaster of emotions and a host of activity centered on autism. Cindy had already processed through fear, anger, denial, bargaining/guilt, and acceptance. She was now entering the stage of resolve, ready to knock down anyone who was in her way. At the moment, it was her husband.

"You've got to be kidding," was all she managed to say after I made the suggestion.

"No, I'm not," I said. "What better way to begin the processing than with some 'take your breath away' sex. Remember that? He needs to be brought on board in a language he understands. And right now his listening ability is down because his 'tank' is empty."

At this point of the story during the panel discussion I was channeling Dr. Ruth. The men in the audience at the conference were yelling "Yeah!" I also heard a man in the front say, "How do I convince my wife that I need to be brought on board more?" It was a free-for-all environment of chaotic laughter as we began to remember how much fun, and how important, sex used to be in our lives. Heck, just talking about it was fun. We used to feel, and be, sexy human beings before autism and responsibilities took over our lives.

I continued the story, telling them that Cindy took my advice and called the next day to say the night of great sex had worked. Her husband had sworn to be more careful with their son's diet. Then she asked for advice on how to get her husband to help with other aspects of their relationship and their child's long-term therapy program.

I told her something that goes completely against our feminist instinct. I suggested she consider really getting his attention. In their case, complete audacity was definitely in order. Pushing her to come out of her comfort zone, I suggested she head down to the local adult store (the one where no one wants to run into anyone they know!) and buy something, then head off to their already scheduled weekend away. Taking clear advantage of this rare opportunity to be alone, I urged her to not talk about the kids, or any heavy concerns on Friday night or Saturday night, but to make her husband her total focus. However, on Sunday morning at breakfast, she was to gently give him a verbal list of the support she needed from him, and to emphasize how crucial his role is in the well-being of their child and family.

The focus-on-the-marriage strategy worked, and Cindy's husband was definitely a happy man too. He even came to one of my talks on dietary intervention. The reality of our lives is that we are more concerned with spending money to get our child well, and less on an expensive B&B weekend away. But the other reality is that we are also more vulnerable to marital discord when our marriage is no longer a priority. The trick is to weave this priority into our stress-filled, cash-strapped lives, and that is our biggest hurdle.

After I related the story about Cindy at the conference, two women came up to me—both with laughter and tears of guilt—recognizing that they had been just like Cindy. One said she now knew how much harder she had made it on herself by fighting her husband, pushing him farther and farther away. She planned to make changes with her husband when she returned from the conference. The other woman approached me with her smiling husband in tow. She too acknowledged that she had been "doing it wrong," and planned to change things that very night. Her husband said he was very happy to hear this. No doubt.

Several women stopped me in the hallway later that day to say, "Girl, you are so right!" They went on to relate stories of how they got their husband's attention in the same way but had not thought about it for autism help. I ran into one of these women six weeks later at another conference. She told me that the strategy had worked wonders in her marriage, and to please write an article about it so that others would know. I did just that.

Acknowledge the Other Person's Need to Grieve

Before sex could ever enter the picture, there had to be an acknowledgement and understanding of the other person's pain and need to grieve. Without understanding how each of us is processing through grief, there is blame and indignation in its place. Many parents facing their child's autism are in personal emotional shutdown.

From my years of mentoring, I noticed that women would tend to process through the grief cycle at a faster pace than men, although not always. Perhaps this was because women were more open with their emotional journeys, making them more likely to come to me for advice or just to talk to someone. But they were also indignant at the perceived emotional shutdown of their husbands. I would explain that, in general, men may need to process through the grief cycle a little longer. They typically want to be supportive of their wives but are often unsure how.

Unfortunately, the many women whom I spoke to were inclined to push their husbands away, put up an emotional wall, and shut down sex. What is not understood by either is that men and women feel equally alone, neglected, and in need of the support of their spouse, especially right after the diagnosis. They are angry at the other for not acknowledging their feelings, believing that the other spouse should change. Both are panicked at the changes in their family and revert to personal survival mode, ostracizing the other spouse in the process. This is when conflict in the marriage is at its worst. Just understanding the cycle of grief for the *temporary* condition that it is may allow couples to focus on the need of their spouse to grieve, and less about chalking up a list of personal grievances that send the marriage into a spiral.

R-E-S-P-E-C-T

Respect is crucial in all discussions about autism-related decisions. But there are times you will want to go to battle with your partner because they are obstinate, or a road block. There is nothing that can be as divisive as deciding how to improve, or overcome, a child's autism. I would like to suggest that this is the time to compromise, but the child will not benefit because compromise takes time. Time really is crucial, and delays in a treatment or therapy can mean a lessening in the progress of what a child may otherwise achieve.

Realistically, not all parents reach a point of agreement on *how* to move forward. One problem can be that parents disagree on the best course of treatment or therapy, although both are equally committed to their child. In some situations that I was involved in, each parent was adamantly convinced that only their own idea would benefit their child. Sometimes a concerned parent worried that the partner's treatment choices might actually harm their child.

I have also seen where the decision-making was really about "control." The need for one parent to control was usually born from a sense of fear. This was certainly true for me. I didn't know what to do for Daniel, so I did everything that seemed reasonable, directing my energy in many directions. If Rich tried to slow me down (really it was s-l-o-w me down) I became panicky over the possibility we might lose precious time. No doubt my fears also fed into the over-the-top stress levels I exuded and endured, to my body's detriment.

In other couples I mentored, one partner was more dominating and the other more of an appeaser. If I picked up that I was speaking with an appeaser, I would say, in so many words, "Wake up, my friend. You need to get engaged in this process. You can no longer take a backseat role. Speak up and make yourself heard because it is your child's future that is at stake." The roles in the marriage are challenged when faced with this situation where the dominator and appeaser have to reverse their tendencies in order to best serve the needs of their child.

Within the quagmire of role reversals is the need to remain respectful of the other parent's opinions. Not enough can be written about the value of *how* we say something, even in the midst of our anxiety-filled decisions. I remember during an argument with Rich, I was shouting the words "I will be treated with dignity and respect at all times!" Of course, I said this while dishing out a lack of respect back at him. Our tone toward each other was something we both had to change if we were going to become a loving couple again.

Timing Is Everything!

If timing is everything, then Silvia, a nervous-sounding, fretful woman, fit the bill of what *not* to do. She asked if it would be okay to bring up her concerns with her husband right after the "fun event" of the evening (her words), believing that after she had done her part it was then time for him to listen to her. Realizing her husband was probably on a perpetual honey-do list at home, I suggested that she back off on any requests for a bit. It is important to understand that he probably felt he had no respite from the worry and crisis she seemed to exude.

This subject is just as important to men. I received an email from a man who read an article I had written. He said he wished he had known sooner what his wife had been going through. He described her as a very successful physician, certain about everything she did except how to help their son. She was feeling vulnerable and tried at times to connect with her husband about her fears. From his perspective, he believed his normally self-assured wife would probably find the answers she needed from her medical colleagues, not him. What he didn't understand was that none of them could replace the emotional support she needed from him. He planned to remedy their emotional disconnect when she came home that night, and hoped that it wasn't too late. I was certain that it wasn't. This is how we begin to reboot our marriages.

Speaking of timing, I like to recommend talking about feelings and concerns during a *quiet* moment (okay, don't choke), as few and far between as these may seem. The key is to really tune in to each other, without the distraction of television, computer, cell phones, or a pile of bills between you. During these times, we are more apt to listen intently to the concerns of our spouse. This practice can go a long way in putting out the flames of bitterness and building a mutual desire to support each other. That quiet moment might be during the child's therapy sessions or while the child is in school, or even a quick phone call from work. Occasionally, we would grab breakfast after dropping off our son at therapy and before Rich went to work. It gave us time to connect with Theresa, who was still young too, while carving a sense of normalcy into our conversation. Just having a cup of coffee together seemed to ease a bit of the disconnect we were feeling.

For me, I had to remember to not barrage Rich with all the complaints of the day right when he walked through the door. There were days when my first instinct was to figure out how bitchy I could sound to him within ten feet of the front door. I learned soon enough that the approach of indignant victimhood just wasn't working for us. Truth is, it doesn't work in any marriage or relationship.

Rich had to be told that budget conversations at ten o'clock at night were strictly forbidden, lest we fall into a worthless argument. My health had taken such a beating from autism-related bad habits that anything that caused stress had to be eliminated, or it would eliminate me. He got the message and pulled back, although, if left up to me, budget conversations would never occur. Autism was enough to deal with.

Go On a Date? Are You Serious?

Oh, the cliché of it all! A date? Are you serious? Sure, and whose reality is that, you ask? *Go on a date?!*

As mentioned, this was us. Dates were for everybody else. Occasionally, we had my mom or sisters babysit, but not for fun evenings out, and certainly not for a dinner that we had to pay for. Even when our son was better we still did not go on dates. Yet, this is what I am suggesting to other couples because we were so far removed from this practice that we forgot how to have fun with each other, and nearly lost our marriage.

If you have one of those fairy grandmothers or other relative who adores all your children, then by all means beg and plead for a night of babysitting. Notify your partner that the night is to be about the two of you. Act like boyfriend and girlfriend and you might actually become that once again. Remember when the excitement of dating was about whether you would have sex later? Wouldn't it be great just to create a little excitement by planning on the sex later?

However, I got a giggle when I heard from a divorced man that he didn't like the idea of sex as a communication tool. For him, it sounded manipulative on the part of the woman. That's when I thought of the dating perspective. First, I acknowledged his concerns from the way I presented it. Then I thought, but didn't say, "You're complaining about sex as a form of manipulation? What's nagging? Isn't that manipulation? For that matter, isn't taking a woman out to dinner a form of manipulation in order to possibly have sex later?" It's all relative. We are just redefining the rules, and we are manipulating the outcome for our marriages. Besides, this is about making the marriage a priority, and sex is a pretty good start to that goal. Going on a date might just make that happen.

It's Okay to Say No

For some couples, the idea of having sex when they are barely speaking, or not even sleeping in the same room, is nearly impossible to imagine. Throw in exhaustion from caring for a child who probably doesn't sleep through the night and the sex idea goes out the window. Start by finding a connection, remembering why you fell in love in the first place. I received an email from a friend that had "Why would I . . .?" as the subject. When I opened the email the only thing written was "have sex with my husband ever again?" I laughed, and then reminded her that she used to dig her husband, back when he was her boyfriend. But it was okay to wait until she felt that connection again. Then I added she could also *fake* it if she was so inclined. Her response to this obvious approach: "LOL!"

One woman in an audience looked at me as if I was from a different planet, as she sat with a pallid face and displayed shell-shocked horror in her body language. I knew the topic of sex as a communication tool was not a reality for her. This is why I encourage men to gently bring their wives through the grief process with an air of confidence, not belligerence. Treat her like a girlfriend, reminding her why you married her in the first place. She may be feeling overwhelmed at the moment and even a bit angry at the burdens forced upon her. There is definitely something positive about the husband taking charge and alleviating the burden, especially if she is not yet ready to cope with decisions. She will take a more active role as she gains her own confidence in the process and in the support she's receiving from her husband.

What needs to be clarified is that no one should feel like a martyr, as though they are put upon or rejected. This approach, meant to encourage communication, should not come with strings attached or with resentment, as if it is an added chore. That's just another form of guilt. Likewise, no one should perpetuate a sense of rejection when their partner does not meet their needs.

When you need help, ask. This is autism, the rules have changed. Even if you are stoic and a hero in all other areas of your life there will come a time when you need help dealing with the crisis. This includes asking for help from your spouse and giving help in return. If a lack of harmony stems from the notion that the other parent "should know what I need," then find the partner's areas of strength and ask for help but don't become focused strictly on what the other person *should* be doing. Not asking, not insisting that your needs are valid means that you have allowed yourself to be used, even if you intend to bear all for the sake of your child. That's false reasoning and may lead to an emergency room visit for you too. When needed, ask for help. If you act like a victim you may become one.

However, it can be tough to go through the process seemingly alone, especially if your partner becomes withdrawn or lashes out. Abuse is never acceptable, nor is shouldering the brunt of the childcare to the point of exhaustion. This is a good time to seek help in all forms, from counseling to respite-care service. If you or your children are being physically abused, this is the time to seek help if necessary, and get out. Let me repeat that in case it is not clear: if you or your children are being abused—get out!

Saying *no* is empowering when it is used to set necessary boundaries and limit unreasonable expectations. For many people who are used to pleasing others, or who have a problem standing up for themselves, the idea of saying no can become a necessary hurdle. Yet, saying no is a measure of freedom. Saying no can also mean that other relationships that interfere with your decisions as a couple must now take a back seat (this is especially true with well-meaning grandparents). Mostly, saying no can also be a way of saying yes to the marriage and family relationships.

Like-Minded Friends Are Your Best Therapists

Someone has got to be around to talk us from the ledge once in a while. I've mentioned the therapy sessions over coffee with like-minded women that got me through the really tough days. These were women who had children with autism too. It was too easy to continuously let our spouses get the blunt end of a very heavy stick when stress levels were through the roof. During our "therapy" sessions over coffee at a restaurant, we would vent our frustrations about our marriages, enough to see that we were not alone in our feelings. We would then laugh at the absurdities and move beyond the angst of our discontent, feeling certain that our individual marriages were in much better shape compared to the others.

I met these women at school pick up lines or at a local support group. We were all going through much of the same discord in our marriages as we all processed through the grief cycle. They weren't always thrilled with my sex idea to process through grief, but they found it fun to talk about sex again, even if it was to talk about how little sex existed in their own marriages. For some men that I mentored, they found it easier to connect with friends outside the autism community because they just wanted to feel normal again, or at least not have autism brought up in a conversation. Whatever way helps to alleviate the strain of the daily burdens is what can lead to better communication at home.

I would suggest a support group to find these like-minded friends, but what I found in my own experiences is that many of these autism groups tend to be pity-parties of those who believe themselves to be victims. If you find a group that empowers and enlightens, then stick with it and hook up with those who are diligently working to help their child and keep their marriages intact. If you don't have such a group in your area, then seek the like-minded friends online. Who knows, you could end up with a new friend across the country who shares your same concerns. I now have a network of friends who only know each other through our journey to get our children well. And we helped each other to get through the worst of days.

Give Each Other Breathing Room

Delilah*, a pretty, petite woman in her thirties, called me up one day when she was upset. Her husband had wanted to go out with his buddies for a weekend of hunting. I couldn't understand why she was so upset until she explained that her whole week was spent taking care of the kids, including her twins with autism. The least he could do was to help her on the weekends.

"So, you guilted him into staying home?" I asked.

"Yes, what else was I supposed to do?" she replied.

With reserved empathy for her plight, I said, "You should have let him go with your blessing. And then at the next opportunity you need to plan a spa weekend away with your girlfriends." I just hope she used the next opportunity to mend this rift in her marriage before real resentment invaded the feelings between them. I understood she was speaking from her exhaustion and frustration of the burdens she had, but there had to be a respite for them both—individually and as a couple.

Giving each other breathing room is a way of acknowledging the other's need to be an individual. By encouraging your partner's hobbies, interests, relationships with friends, desire to be healthy and desire to go have fun, you are creating a sense of intimacy without being intimate. At the same time, expect the same for yourself. Working together to create independent alone time is another way to encourage the relationship's growth and harmony through the tough times. This is what helps us connect again, both as individuals and as a couple. Breathing room gives us respite from the crisis and shores up our ability to endure our daily demands. It also reminds us that we are valuable as individuals too.

Expect Bad Days

There will be days when your child's behavior leaves you with nothing to give, especially to your partner. Just understanding this fact alone can alleviate the notion that one bad day makes it one bad marriage. Coming to terms with this reality forced me to consciously change my focus to one of "deep appreciation" for my husband (alternating with rage at a moment's notice!). It was the effort to change what *I* could do that made all the difference. It was easier to change my outlook than it was to change my husband. It took a while, but I believe my husband finally came to the same conclusion about me.

Above all else, don't buy into the myths that surround the divorce rates in the autism community as though that is your destiny. For years, it was presumed, or even predetermined, that most families with a child who has autism would eventually fall under the umbrella of "divorced" or "separated." The myth that permeated the autism community was that we experienced a sky-high divorce rate of eighty percent. As a mentor to these families, I knew this figure was wrong because I didn't see this level of divorce. I saw couples sticking together because they could not afford to divorce or could not bear to care for their child with autism alone. At least those are the reasons they gave during our conversation. Perhaps it also was because they were still in love and not sure how to get back on track yet.

Finally, researchers from the Kennedy Krieger Institute in Maryland were able to debunk a lot of the misunderstandings about high divorce rates among parents of autistic children. In their extensive study published in 2010, they found that sixty-four percent of children with an autism spectrum disorder (ASD) belonged to a family with two married biological or adoptive parents, compared with sixty-five percent of children who do not have autism. In other words, there was very little difference between families who had children with autism and those that did not. One factor that was not mentioned was the health of the autism-family marriages. Were they happy or in a state of constant marital strife? As I read this study, I wanted to add in the obvious: *all* of our marriages were going through, or about to go through, hell. The reason was grief, and these were the bad days. It's just that these bad days were not necessarily going to permanently damage our marriages as long as we didn't allow it to happen.

If we understood the impact of grief upon marriages, the parents in the autism community might finally stop selling themselves, and their marriages, short. Their marriages are not failing. They are enduring difficult days, even difficult years. It's just a matter of time (preferably not too long) for the process of grief to be complete, and then the real healing in the marriage can begin.

Meditate and Pray

It may not be for everyone, but some sort of giving in to a Higher Power can help extinguish the hardness of hearts and reshape conversations to be more positive and loving. Over time, the very act of focusing on a Higher Source can begin to mend the marriage and keep it intact. Some couples attend church, temple, or mosque together and find a connection that way. For others that is not a part of their lives. It can also be an individual choice that can positively impact the marriage.

I like to meditate to calm my stress levels and to keep my sanity in check. However, Rich and I are more individualistic with our method of praying and asking for spiritual help. I remember begging God to please guide me to find the answers in order to save our son. If Rich did the same, I never heard about it. I assumed he prayed because we were both fighting for our son and pulling out all of the stops. I have to believe he prayed for us too.

A deity, of course, is not necessary in order to relinquish control within the mind for a brief period. When I speak with groups, I often recommend meditation, even if it is only five minutes. The only thing I tell them is that the time they "zone out" is to be used to clear their minds, not go through their mental checklist of everything they have to do that day. I also tell them to not use it as a grievance session, a time to add up all of the worries and hurt feelings plaguing them at the time. If you just check out mentally for a little while, chances are you will become addicted to the sense of mental and internal clarity that happens during meditation. Do it enough times and even the worries about the marriage improve, and our thinking about what to do to help our children becomes clearer.

Breaking Up Is Hard to Do

Let's face it, not all marriages are going to survive autism. Even before autism hits, many are on the edge and need only one more stressor to finally convince them that their humpty-dumpty marriage is over. In cases like this, autism may be the final reason for why a couple chooses to divorce. Ideally, the parents are in some kind of agreement on the need for their child to receive the right treatments and therapies. Once they agree that treatment in necessary, the expense of possible therapies becomes the next hurdle. Their combined incomes are now down to single-parent status. I typically coach the parents to focus on what they *can* do financially. If diet is the issue, then food needs to be stored at both houses. I've often heard from one parent about having to supply the food for the non-custodial parent since the other parent "did not want to be bothered" by an alternative diet.

When I mentor divorced couples, I find it best to speak with each parent separately, passing along identical information. Invariably, some couples harbor such resentment toward the other that they cannot focus on their child. A young, single mother came up to me after a presentation on this topic and said she enjoyed it, but wondered what to do about dating while caring for the child with autism. That is a tough one because we all know how difficult our day is with our child. If you find a person willing to work with you through the bad days, then please hold on to him or her. But in the end, you are still the parent who needs to make decisions for the sake of your child.

Charlotte*, another single mother in her thirties, asked a question about her fiancé's reaction to how she disciplined her son versus how his daughter was disciplined. He felt she applied a double standard because her son had autism and was not disciplined at all. I told the mother that I saw his point. Realistic expectations must be set for her son. If her son could understand consequences, then she needed to step up the discipline for him. I'm not sure Charlotte totally agreed with me but this man was marrying into a tough situation. A doable compromise would help them create their new family.

What's the Goal?

The man and woman sitting in the front row nodded in eager agreement as I spoke about how autism changes marriages. Rather than give in to the daunting statistic of how eighty percent of our marriages were doomed to fail, I outlined how they were destined to improve their marriages by overcoming this difficult time in their lives with a stronger union to show for it. Certain that my message to this audience had hit home with a marriage or two saved, I was stunned when the couple in the front row told the audience that they were already divorced. They also decided they would not have divorced the year before if they had heard this discussion about grief and marriage earlier. They had bought into the belief of autism ruining their marriage but came to a new realization that very night. Their casual hand touch said it all. They would find a new way to help their family survive autism, together.

The goal is to achieve *normalcy* in our families—however we define that word—every day of our very un-normal lives. For me, it was remembering why I fell in love with Rich in the first place. He can find humor in the most absurd of situations, and I am his best audience because I laugh at all of his jokes. Our daughter also had to be reminded how important she is to us. We gave her one-on-one time to ensure that she felt just as special as her brother. We even took time to treat Daniel to individual time with each of us, creating a bond with him that had nothing to do with a therapy session. And, as a family, we made it a point to bond together in the simple and even mundane moments.

But it all began with the bond between Rich and me. Our family survived, even thrived with autism, with our marriage and family intact. I just need to convince Rich that an expensive B&B weekend away is still a good idea. And he will have to convince me that lingerie is worth the effort. No matter, I am still his sexy girlfriend and he is the guy who still takes my breath away. At least we now remember who we used to be.

Chapter Six

My Brother's/Sister's Keeper: Fostering the Needs of the Typical Sibling

It was going to be a blowout birthday party; well, as far as a birthday for a three-year-old is concerned. The birthday girl had been through a rough year. Her younger brother had been diagnosed with autism a year before and her mother and father were in high gear to meet his needs. The little girl was part of every doctor's appointment and therapy session, and affected by her parents' constant focus on her brother's needs. She took it all in stride in a way that seemed to belie her young age, as though she secretly knew that what was going on with her brother was important.

That little girl was Theresa. Looking back, it is hard to imagine how any child could have endured the level of stress Rich and I were projecting as we sought answers for Daniel. But Theresa did, and in many ways she kept us all balanced, even as a two-year-old.

But, as her mother, I needed my little girl to know how important she was to us too, so I began to plan her third birthday party two months in advance. Besides, it was also a distraction from the mindless anxiety I was otherwise gravitating to, and something fun to do. The theme was "Wizard of Oz" since it was the one movie she watched over and over, singing and skipping right along with Dorothy. I even found a woman to come dressed as Dorothy who brought an entire themed entertainment session with her, playing "Somewhere over the Rainbow" on the boom box as she came into the party. The look on Theresa's face was priceless. She knew the day was all about her and she would never forget it. To this day, she says that her third birthday was the one she would never forget as it was her favorite.

When she was fifteen months old, she spoke her first full sentence: "Mama, don't touch the baby." It was something I must have repeated a dozen times to her in that first month after her brother was born. The funny thing is she said it with a sense that her baby brother was hers to look after, and in many ways that is exactly what she did. There were times when Rich and I would shake our heads in amazement at how they got along as brother and sister, in a way that neither of us did with our own siblings. Part of their relationship is nothing we could have taught them, but something they fostered on their own.

Still, I worried that all of the attention on Daniel would somehow limit the attention Theresa received, and maybe resentment toward her brother would set in. I had reason to worry about this as I watched the families of older children deal with this dichotomy in their own families.

"My son feels that his brother ruined his life. He hates him, and I can understand why. But it doesn't make it any easier for any of us." That was the conversation I had with a woman whose teenage son was overwhelmed and fed up with the demands of time and energy that his younger brother's behaviors had on the family. While the parents worked to calm the younger child, the older child was often left to deal with the grief and anger from the loss of a "normal" childhood.

Conversely, there are the children who find purpose and joy in their role as their sibling's playmate, helper, and therapist. They are often protective, and become staunch advocates for the sibling that may one day be in their care. The difference between the two family situations may be found in the grief cycle, and how each child is allowed to process through these emotions. These are the generation of children who will more than likely be the eventual guardians of their siblings when their parents no longer can. How do we help these vital members of the family overcome their own sense of loss of a "normal" childhood?

The Child's Grief Cycle

By the time Theresa was fifteen, she had five friends who had lost a parent due to death. Some of those friends were close enough that the grief process happened while they were around us, and we helped them to feel safe enough to express their grief, even crying with them. On a couple of occasions, I would illustrate to the surviving parent how the grief cycle would possibly play out, encouraging one of Theresa's friends to move past the pain by allowing herself to go through it instead of shutting down and choosing to ignore it. She eventually did and finally began to heal.

At a recent funeral of a young man, I overheard a family member tell the deceased's eight-year-old son that he was now the "man of the house" and should therefore not cry. The boy quickly wiped away his tears, took a deep breath and tried to compose himself. But it was too much to ask of anyone, let alone an eight year old who was now fatherless, and the pain shook his young body all over again.

Loss redefines us, even when we don't think it ever will. As children, the loss redefines what we think of ourselves and our place in the world. With typical siblings of the children with autism, their loss of the childhood routine is defined within how the rest of us define "normal." With autism, the family dynamic is altered, and the sibling is left to possibly grieve their own sense of loss—or not. How each child processes through grief is determined by factors that lend toward how the child feels about themselves and their place in their world.

Years ago I was listening to a radio talk show host doling out advice to a father of a child with autism. Apparently, this man told the host that his typical daughter was so resentful toward her brother that she took to hitting him when the parents were not around. The girl was ten and knew better. As the father explained, his daughter was frustrated toward her brother because it affected how she was perceived by her friends. She hated his behaviors and all of the energy he took up in the house.

The father assured the talk show host that the daughter received sufficient attention and had been told the hitting was unacceptable. The host then told the father that the next course of action was to give this young girl a spanking. I was shocked. Not in my wildest thoughts did the notion of spanking ever cross my mind as a remedy for this behavior. All over the US there were parents shouting into the radio. NO! What this girl was doing was not acceptable, but it was understandable. What the father failed to mention was the fact that this boy, through no fault of his own, deprived her of an ordinary childhood, thereby redefining the family dynamic.

You see, the parents are not the only ones who need to go through a period of grieving. It can also happen to the other children. They mourn the loss of the sibling relationship and they mourn having to feel like a "different" kind of family. Helping this child to grasp her grief would have been a better course of action. I sincerely hoped this father did not take the advice of the spanking and instead sought the help of a seasoned counselor to guide the family through grief and to meet the needs of every family member.

Creating That Balance

"Tiffany is really upset at me," said the young mother during a tearful phone conversation. "She thinks I don't love her like Trevor." She then went on to tell me that her six-year-old daughter had said something that left the mother speechless. Apparently, the mother had a habit of speaking in a baby tone with her son, who was just a year younger than her daughter. This bothered the little girl very much. When she asked her mother why she spoke in this endearing tone with her brother and not with her, the mother had no answer.

After the mother told me the story, I asked her when the last time it was that she went out with her daughter as just the two of them, even to get ice cream. You could tell this well-intentioned mother felt bad; she had so singularly put her focus on her son's tenuous health that her daughter was clearly not getting the attention she needed or deserved. Besides the obvious benefit to her daughter, the mom also needed a little "girl time." It made me realize how easy it was to get tunnel vision for the sake of our child with special needs, and lose sight of the necessary balance.

I have also seen the opposite, where the child with autism is virtually ignored in favor of the activities of the other children. One family marginalized the needs of their child with autism to the point that any treatments for him were weighed against the sports needs of the other children. He sat in the bleachers at their games perseverating with an electronic device.

Parents are essential to ensuring that the typical child feels like they are valued members of the family. When Daniel was dropped off at physical therapy, Theresa and I would carve out that brief time to have some girl time at a local café, where she ordered a treat and I had a cup of coffee while we "chatted" about anything she wanted to talk about. It cemented the nature of our relationship, even in the teen years, when she still found it easy to turn to me to talk about whatever was on her mind because we always have. Her dad also made it a point to take her out to special places just to have his time with his girl.

So too with Daniel, it mattered to have time together that had nothing to do with autism. A friend of mine told me how her son had begged her to not do therapy for a single day so that he had the time to play. This mom was excellent at researching all of the latest techniques, therapies, and treatments and implemented everything she thought would benefit her son. He absolutely improved, but the one-sided focus meant that her young son was now begging for time to just be a kid. I tossed in the idea that she cancel all appointments the next day and head off to a local theme park, just the two of them. I don't know if they did, but the idea was planted to allow for the normal to enter the lives of our children—and the parent. This idea of a single fully-child-focused day is good for the other children as well. We have since made it a habit to find time to have fun that has nothing to do with expectations or schedules.

One mother related that her six-year-old son was often hurt and confused when his younger brother with autism refused to play with him or engage in any sort of activity, except on rare occasions. To make the older boy not feel bad about being pushed away by his brother, the parents used the analogy that the younger brother was like Spiderman, with "tingly" senses, and that it was up to the older brother to help Spiderman find his way in the world. It was a duty the older boy took seriously since he could relate to the idea of Spiderman having "tingly" senses.

Another parent had two teenage sons, the typical son being slightly older than his sibling. While he loved his younger brother the interaction between them was difficult because his brother was non-verbal and his behaviors dictated how the family made plans of any kind. And since he felt awkward and conspicuous because of his brother's behaviors, he would not dare invite friends over. When the older boy started high school he began to play football, which seemed to be exactly the outlet he needed to begin forging friendships. His father was thrilled as he longed to have this kind of bonding opportunity with his son. I heard later that the father became head of the local Football Booster Club, and the father and son bonded as they never had before. This helped ease the tension the older boy had toward his brother because he no longer felt like his brother was blocking his effort to fit in.

An acquaintance mentioned how her younger son had many friends and was invited out a lot. His older brother with Asperger's felt left out, even though he normally avoided social situations. This was difficult for the mother to watch. She was not going to impede her younger son's social growth, but she worried about how it was affecting her older son, emotionally. Instead of placating her older son with platitudes she made it a point instead to encourage his effort to seek out friends of his own.

We have had this happen at times between Theresa and Daniel. While Theresa made friends easily, Daniel's friends were fewer and not as available. We knew the development of normal relationships with peers had to be done from their own efforts, not ours, even if all we did to help it along is create the opportunity to connect with peers. This happens in many families, not just special needs. While we encouraged Daniel's effort, we did not intervene. For other children, however, this is exactly the area they need the most help, which is why they often attach themselves to the typical child as a sole playmate.

Siblings Need Respite, Too

Just as parents need an occasional respite from the daily care of their special needs child, so too does the typical child need to step away from the daily interaction with their sibling. Even when a child is considered *mild*, the impact can be felt by the other children. One family I know used to schedule days for their oldest child to be away from the younger sibling just to give the older girl a break from having to be with her sister as a sole playmate. The younger girl had fewer friends and therefore sought out her sister. As a child, my father was the only playmate for his older, mentally disabled sister. He believes it may have stifled his own social interaction with boys his own age.

As a young mother prepared her eight-year-old daughter for a vacation away from her family, the look of anticipation was greater with the mother, it seemed, than her daughter. The mother recognized that her daughter was under stress from the day-to-day activities surrounding her younger brother and she reached out to her family to see if they would take her daughter for a couple of weeks of respite care—preferably with lots of spoiling for a girl that seemed to be in desperate need of individual attention. Her grandmother and aunts took up the duty with gusto and pleasure, certain that their task was a win-win for everyone. As it was, the girl was entirely the focus of attention from all of the relatives, which seemed to fill the tank, and she was ready to come home at the end of the two weeks, completely satisfied.

My sister-in-law hosted her cousin's daughter for two weeks many years ago when we all lived in California. The girl had a brother with severe autism, leaving the mother of the children exhausted and entirely focused on his physical needs. It was a welcome break for the girl to step away even for a couple of weeks to focus on herself.

More than One Child on the Spectrum

I have met families with three, four, and five children with spectrum disorders. What is common in families who have at last one child with autism is that one or multiple siblings have autism or other related disorders like ADD, ADHD, OCD, or even bipolar. As the parents balance the physical needs of each child they are then left to pull together the threads of a loving relationship with each child, and then to help their children foster it with each other.

One family I met had five children, three of whom had autism. Two of the children with autism were "runners" at night, attempting to run outdoors into traffic. The parents would take turns sleeping downstairs just to avoid a catastrophe. The impact on the other two children was daunting. These brave parents did all they could to maintain a sense of normalcy by encouraging the typical children to foster friendships and activities outside the home, while still participating in their lives as parents.

Long ago, my husband and I knew a family who had three children with special needs, all different in complexity. The father joked that they didn't have "normal" children, which caused me to flinch because the term can be used in a derogatory manner. He didn't mean it that way, of course, but it was clear this family faced a challenge at balancing all their needs.

A dear friend has two sons with autism, who are now grown, with the older one being more affected by autism than his younger brother. It was interesting to watch how the mother would guide each one according to their abilities, including the older one getting his driver's license. Even with the same diagnosis they both presented with different needs, so it was a matter of juggling the emotional, social, and physical needs of each. It became even more complex when they became adults and were beginning to navigate some moments of independence, with each proving to be more capable, or more challenged, in different areas.

The Community is Ready to Talk about This Important Issue

This topic of how autism affects the siblings is huge in the autism community. There is no formal organized program to support the siblings except occasional workshops called Sibshops, which are leading the way in addressing the social and emotional needs of siblings of special needs children.

What needs to be done is to make this more holistic in scope. Picture this: as of this moment, when I am writing this chapter, there is an autism rate of 1 in 68 in the US. But we in the autism community know that the number is much higher since we see it in our schools, on the playgrounds, and everywhere else we turn. The numbers of children being diagnosed is an epidemic in the United States, even if the CDC will not admit that fact yet. And with every child diagnosed there is a high probability a sibling will reel from the impact on their childhood, too.

Lisa R. wrote to tell me that this topic hit close to home. Her daughter felt so alone from having a brother with autism that her mother set up an Edmodo group for her to connect with other girls her age who were going through the same thing. When Lisa returned from an autism conference, her young daughter decided it was her turn to go to get support and came out with a packed bag to say she was ready to leave. It dawned on Lisa then how much her daughter had internalized and how much she too needed to be supported, just as Lisa was. So she helped her daughter to start the Edmodo support group to connect with other siblings, who all needed to know it was okay and that they were not alone.

It may be an element of tough love mixed with pragmatism that led Lisa to later firmly tell her daughter that "life is not fair; we all get dealt with stuff." Lisa said that, as a military family, they had gotten really good at adapting. Still, Lisa worried that the troubles associated with being the "second child" would follow her into adolescence and beyond.

"I try to undo her negative self-talk," Lisa explained. "She is the 'normal' kid in the family so she is feeling the pressure. No one expects her to, but she puts this sense of perfection on herself." She went on to say that she had her daughter in therapy too.

Another mother wrote in saying that her daughter also felt left out because her days were filled with her brother's therapy and doctor appointments. The mother lamented that at a time when her daughter's friends were heading out to dance lessons or girl scouts, her own daughter could not because the mother had to focus on the immediate physical needs of her son.

Conversely, a close friend told the story of how her young son with autism was dropped off to therapy, giving her and her slightly older son a chance to browse Target and pick up small toys for just him. But one day the older boy began to cry in the middle of the store. When his mother was able to calm him down she asked him what was wrong, and he told her that he wanted to play too. He had concluded that his younger brother was given privileges of "play" and that as the oldest he was not allowed to participate. The mother had to assure him that his brother's "play sessions" were actually to help him become better. It helped the older boy to understand, but he still felt a pang of regret from the thought that he was being left out.

Lisa Ackerman sent me a blog post on this topic that she wrote titled "The Forgotten Children," which spotlighted the impact autism has on our other children, using as an example how her own teenage daughter reacted when Lisa became solely focused on her son's needs:

> After a tough day at school, Lauren came into the room and told me she really needed to talk to me. I knew it was going to be about some drama because she's sixteen and in high school. So she went on to tell me how everyone sucks and yada yada yada and I said to her, "Lauren, I don't care what your friend said. I don't care what happened at your school today. You've got that bitchy sixteen-year-old look on your face about some friend telling you something that hurt your feelings. I really don't care." She looked at me for a moment and started crying. Then she said, "You know, you have two kids, Mom."
>
> My world stopped. This is the other moment in my life where I died a little bit inside. I had nothing for anyone but Jeff. I became this single-focused person that no one wanted to live with. I didn't even want to live with me. I tried to think back to the time when I was a nurturing, fun mom who gave Lauren what she needed. That is who I wanted to be again.

Most emails I receive on this topic include the word "guilt," which is generally attached to the parents' sense of it as they wrestle with securing services and treatments for their child with autism while trying to care for the emotional, social, and physical needs of the typical child. It's a balancing act that few of us master.

Natalie Palumbo—A Sister's Story

By the time she was fourteen years old, Natalie Palumbo had decided she would one day be her brother's caregiver. Now a motion design major at Ringling University in Florida, Natalie forthrightly declares that her older brother Anthony is her past, present, and, most important, future priority. She says it with such determination that there is no doubt she knows that she and Anthony are joined at the hip, intertwined in such a way that all of Natalie's dating relationships know that she and Anthony are a package deal.

While some siblings may consider lifelong care of a sibling to be a daunting prospect, Natalie has welcomed the idea to the point that her future career and family plans all have Anthony in the picture. In her mind, she is not the least bit noble about her stance, just doing the right thing to make sure he is never abused or mistreated by anyone. That, to her, is more daunting than the idea of taking care of her brother.

When Natalie was a senior in high school she made her first PSA film about autism, detailing what autism actually is, not the myths and general impressions people think it is. She made the film in part because of her own fears of the lack of services for older children who were aging out of the system. It's part of Natalie's nature to worry about her brother. She watched him have severe allergic reactions to foods and medicines over the years, and be abused by typical peers. It was heartbreaking to Natalie to know her sweet brother could be abused by anyone, let alone kids his own age. This is why she made the PSA and geared it to a younger audience so that they would understand the real nature of autism.

Natalie is simultaneously open about her brother while remaining somewhat cautious with what she talks about when he is the subject. She is his staunchest advocate and protector and it's a task she does not take lightly.

"He has always been the most important person to me," says Natalie with a certainty that belies her youth. She can then describe how her parents encouraged her to speak about her feelings and concerns while growing up, and brought her into the fold of information as it pertained to what was going on with her brother. This is probably why she understands what foods he reacts to and medications he cannot handle, as well as other medical issues that usually only rest within the knowledge of the parents. For Natalie, her parents made her a partner in this knowledge, in part because she wanted to know.

When she began her college life and began to make career goals, every decision was weighed against how she would achieve her primary goal of being able to provide and care for her brother in the future.

"I want to know he is safe. I want to be able to live comfortably with him. Some siblings are resentful. In my case, I don't want to see anything bad happen to him," says Natalie as a way of making her point clear on her future plans.

Taking care of Anthony was not an expectation imposed by her parents, but rather a calling from within Natalie. And the relationship she has with her brother can only be described as remarkable. They seem to always be looking out for each other, with Anthony finding trinkets to buy his sister on his excursions, and Natalie creating videos specifically for her brother's enjoyment. Natalie credits her parents for giving her a voice through her childhood, by listening to her and validating her contribution as a member of the family. She recognizes that not all siblings of special needs children have been afforded the same relationship in their families, and grow up with a sense of jealousy and resentment.

She went through a period of grief over her brother's autism when it hit her that it was unlikely that he would ever recover from autism. She reflects that she was fourteen or fifteen years old when the realization hit her. Later, she would discuss her desire to have her brother recover from autism and was at times faced with accusations by others that she must not love her brother enough since she wanted to "change" him. This hurt and infuriated her because the reality of autism is that her brother could not communicate his needs and was often sick. Yes, she wanted recovery—for Anthony's sake! But even without it, Natalie will continue to be his best friend. And he, hers.

The Therapists' Turn . . .

Many of the therapists who work with families of special needs have a calling to the profession, often because they also have a family member with special needs and feel united in the plights of the clients they serve. One such therapist is Jonah Green, a licensed certified social worker and therapist who runs Jonah Green and Associates out of Kensington, Maryland. He specializes in families with special needs children, with a strong emphasis on the entire family dynamic. While he likes to focus first on the relationship between the parents, he has also worked holistically to include the needs of the siblings.

"I work to form a family perspective, including multiple family members at a time," explains Jonah. "I have found that, oftentimes, everyone has their own therapist and that is not always the most useful way of addressing this. Someone needs to have a view of the family as a whole, and that as individuals they are getting their needs met."

"There is an overall strain on the individuals to getting their needs met, and certain relationships getting their needs met. There may be feelings of annoyance toward the sibling [with disabilities], being the kid who gets more attention from parents. So there is anger, jealousy, and kinds of feelings like embarrassment," explained Jonah. The problem is made worse when imbalances create alliances that are cross-generational, like a parent and sibling teaming up against the other parent and special needs sibling. This pattern sets off a domino effect of dysfunction in the family that needs to be dealt with head on in order to put relationship balance back into the family unit.

Many typical siblings face being ostracized from their peers because autism can be viewed as contagious even from a social stigma perspective. He also related that typical siblings can either be stigmatized by their special needs brother or sister, or be invigorated. Jonah continues to explain that siblings often develop core strengths. They learn flexibility, tolerance for differences, and empathy. But this happens only after the developmentally healthy needs of the typical child are met.

He circles it back to the relationship with the parents because once that relationship is healthy then they can nurture the needs of the children accordingly. Each person has their needs met, has a constructive role in the family, and has a bond with the parent. This is the road toward improving the family relationships. Jonah also suggested that siblings need to work out their own relationship without interference from the parents, something he acknowledges is more difficult with a special needs child, but still relevant to helping them form and build their own bond.

Sarah Norris is a hippotherapist, a form of physical therapy that uses horseback riding. She works at the Bridge Center in Bridgewater, Massachusetts, serving individuals with special needs. Her own life is a mirror of the lives many of siblings of her clients are experiencing, only with a few differences. Her older brother has special needs, currently under the guardianship of her parents. The one thing Sarah is most grateful for is that her parents made key decisions to plan for the long term well-being of her older brother, and made sure that Sarah and her middle brother understood the plans they had made and what their roles would be once the parents passed on. That kind of planning took the pressure off of Sarah and her middle brother, with the latter destined to be his brother's guardian at some point.

However, many of the siblings of the children she serves are very aware of the difficulties that lie before them; with many worried enough that they make their own life plans around the needs of their disabled sibling. Some are so jealous and resentful over the impact their sibling had on their own childhood that they forego any contact once they reach adulthood. But Sarah and others discovered that the siblings are the ones who are most connected. They know more things about their brother or sister than any of the adults in their lives, including their parents.

There is a part of being a sibling that parents cannot appreciate. They have an interesting perspective on their sibling while parents are focused on therapy, Sarah explained. "They are the expert on their sibling and see them as another kid," Sarah said.

She began to conduct Sibshops through her organization where it was decided to bring both the special needs and their typical siblings together in a fun environment. Most Sibshops are done strictly for the typical child to give them a place that did not include their special needs sibling. But Sarah believed it important that the typical children be allowed to come together with their special needs sibling, and bond separately with their peers. The typical children were able to see that other children their age had siblings with special needs, and that they (the typical children) were not alone. They didn't just talk about it. They could meet each other's siblings through the camp program, which included horseback riding for all of them. They still bonded as peers and then bonded separately with each other's siblings. Sarah said that some of the typical children were very excited to see what their siblings were doing at camp, and others truly wanted no involvement with their special needs sibling.

Don Meyer is the founder and Director of the Sibling Support Project. He is also the founder of the SEFAM (Supporting Extended Family Members) program at the University of Washington, which pioneered services for fathers, siblings, and grandparents of children with special needs. He is the creator and founder of Sibshops through the Sibling Support Project. When Don began the entire concept of Sibshops in 1990, he had no idea that a quarter of a century later he would be the only person in the US who worked full time to address the needs of the siblings. While there were scores of full-time workers dedicated to the parents and children with special needs, there were very few who were trying to bring the siblings through the continuous crisis in their lives, and give them a voice.

"If you support, inform, validate, and celebrate (the sibling), they will increase the chances to remain involved with the siblings when the parents are no longer around," remarked Don. It's his passion, his calling, to instill in the broader community the need to provide for the sibling their own voice, encouraging their individuality in the process.

"I know siblings that are conceived with a job description," said Don, suggesting that for some families there is this underlying expectation that a typical sibling will one day be the sole caregiver for their disabled brother or sister. "They need to know they have everybody's blessing to have a life of their own," he added. It is in this dynamic that Don has dedicated himself to increasing the understanding and awareness of the needs of the typical child. He is the author or editor of six books dealing with the needs of the family members, especially the siblings of special needs children.

Sibshops were set up to help these "underserved" members of the family feel they are not alone and that they matter. The workshops are designed to be fun outlets in a relaxed environment, allowing the children to naturally connect with others without a sense of formality. "We talk about things but it is not therapy," Don explained. He elaborated that the contributions of the siblings are spotlighted and they are reminded that the session is about them.

Don echoed what Sarah said about the siblings having a unique perspective of their siblings, suggesting they are usually fairly accurate in what the sibling with special needs was capable of doing on their own. He said that the families of the most adjusted typical children are the ones that didn't treat the child with special needs as incapable, or any more special than the other children. "In our family Tim was just another kid," Don remarks as an example of an older sibling who felt that his needs were met growing up.

Another example demonstrated how the typical child believed the sibling with special needs was more capable than the parents did. "I wish they made my sister do what I knew she could do," said the typical child of their sibling with autism. Don shared other examples of how a typical child perceived their sibling's limitations versus capabilities. It also fell in line with how the typical child perceived him or herself, and their role in the family.

The main component of the support groups is to echo what parents intuitively hope for themselves—to not feel alone on the journey. And that is what Don is trying to capture with every training lecture he gives on the whole concept of Sibshops. When he wrote *What Siblings Want Every Parent and Service Provider to Know,* he did so with the understanding that this segment of the population was growing significantly. The siblings would be the ones involved with their brother or sister over their life span, longer even than the parents. What was being done to address their needs?

Don clarifies, "Brothers and sisters, often left in the literal and figurative waiting rooms of service delivery systems, deserve better. True family-centered care and services will arrive when siblings are actively included in an agency's functional definition of 'family.'"

The following is what Don wrote on the subject. I put it in its entirety with his permission because it spotlights the needs of the siblings fully. It's a movement that needs to catch fire in our community, and it is about time.

What Siblings Want Every Parent and Service Provider to Know, by Don Meyer

1. **The Right to One's Own Life.**

   Throughout their lives, brothers and sisters may play many different roles in the lives of their siblings who have special needs. Regardless of the contributions they may make, the basic right of siblings to their own lives must always be remembered. Parents and service providers should not make assumptions about responsibilities typically-developing siblings may assume without a frank and open discussion. "Nothing about us without us"—a phrase popular with self-advocates who have disabilities—applies to siblings as well. Self-determination, after all, is for everyone—including brothers and sisters.

2. **Acknowledging Siblings' Concerns.**

   Like parents, brothers and sisters will experience a wide array of often ambivalent emotions regarding the impact of their siblings' special needs. These feelings should be both expected and acknowledged by parents and other family members and service providers. Because most siblings will have the longest-lasting relationship with the family member who has a disability, these concerns will change over time. Parents and providers would be wise to learn more about siblings' life-long and ever-changing concerns.

3. **Expectations for Typically-Developing Siblings.**

   Families need to set high expectations for all their children. However, some typically-developing brothers and sisters react to their siblings' disability by setting unrealistically high expectations for themselves—and some feel that they must somehow compensate for their siblings' special needs. Parents can help their typically-developing children by conveying clear expectations and unconditional support.

4. Expect Typical Behavior from Typically-Developing Siblings.

Although difficult for parents to watch, teasing, name-calling, arguing, and other forms of conflict are common among most brothers and sisters—even when one has special needs. While parents may be appalled at siblings' harshness toward one another, much of this conflict can be a beneficial part of normal social development. A child with Down syndrome who grows up with siblings with whom he sometimes fights will likely be better prepared to face life in the community as an adult than a child with Down syndrome who grows up as an only child. Regardless of how adaptive or developmentally appropriate it might be, typical sibling conflict is more likely to result in feelings of guilt when one sibling has special health or developmental needs. When conflict arises, the message sent to many brothers and sisters is, "Leave your sibling alone. You are bigger, you are stronger, you should know better. It is your job to compromise." Typically-developing siblings deserve a life where they, like other children, sometimes misbehave, get angry, and fight with their siblings.

5. Expectations for the Family Member with Special Needs.

When families have high expectations for their children who have special needs, everyone will benefit. As adults, typically-developing brothers and sisters will likely play important roles in the lives of their siblings who have disabilities. Parents can help siblings now by helping their children who have special needs acquire skills that will allow them to be as independent as possible as adults. To the extent possible, parents should have the same expectations for the child with special needs regarding chores and personal responsibility as they do for their typically-developing children. Not only will similar expectations foster independence, it will also minimize the resentment expressed by siblings when there are two sets of rules—one for them, and another for their sibs who have special needs.

6. **The Right to a Safe Environment.**

Some siblings live with brothers and sisters who have challenging behaviors. Other siblings assume responsibilities for themselves and their siblings that go beyond their age level and place all parties in vulnerable situations. Siblings deserve to have their own personal safety given as much importance as the family member who has special needs.

7. **Opportunities to Meet Peers.**

For most parents, the thought of "going it alone," raising a child with special needs without the benefit of knowing another parent in a similar situation would be unthinkable. Yet, this routinely happens to brothers and sisters. Sibshops, listservs such as SibNet and SibKits, and similar efforts offer siblings the common-sense support and validation that parents get from parent-to-parent programs and similar programs. Brothers and sisters—like parents—like to know that they are not alone with their unique joys and concerns.

8. **Opportunities to Obtain Information.**

Throughout their lives, brothers and sisters have an ever-changing need for information about their sibling's disability, and its treatment and implications. Parents *and* service providers have an obligation to proactively provide siblings with helpful information. Any agency that represents a specific disability or illness and prepares materials for parents and other adults should prepare materials for siblings and young readers as well.

9. **Sibs' Concerns about the Future.**

Early in life, many brothers and sisters worry about what obligations they will have toward their sibling in the days to come. Ways parents can reassure their typically-developing children are to make plans for the future of their children with special needs, involve and listen to their typically-developing children as they make these plans, consider backup plans, and know that siblings' attitude toward the extent of their involvement as adults may change over time.

When brothers and sisters are "brought into the loop" and given the message early that they have their parents' blessing to pursue their dreams, their future involvement with their sibling will be a choice instead of an obligation. For their own good and for the good of their siblings who have disabilities, brothers and sisters should be afforded the right to their own lives. This includes having a say in whether and how they will be involved in the lives of their siblings who have disabilities as adults, and the level, type, and duration of involvement.

10. Including Both Sons and Daughters.

Just as daughters are usually the family members who care for aging parents, adult sisters are usually the family members who look after the family member with special needs when the parents no longer can. Serious exploration of sharing responsibilities among siblings—including brothers—should be considered.

11. Communication.

While good communication between parents and children is always important, it is especially important in families where there is a child who has special needs. An evening course in active listening can help improve communication among all family members, and books, such as *How to Talk So Kids Will Listen and Listen So Kids Will Talk* and *Siblings without Rivalry* (both by Adele Faber and Elaine Mazlich) provide helpful tips on communicating with children.

12. One-on-One Time with Parents.

Children need to know from their parents' deeds and words that their parents care about them as individuals. When parents carve time out of a busy schedule to grab a bite at a local burger joint or window shop at the mall with their typically-developing children, it conveys a message that parents "are there" for them as well and provides an excellent opportunity to talk about a wide range of topics.

13. Celebrate Every Child's Achievements and Milestones.

Over the years, we've met siblings whose parents did not attend their high school graduation—even when their children were valedictorians—because the parents were unable to leave their child with special needs. We've also met siblings whose wedding plans were dictated by the needs of their sibling who had a disability. One child's special needs should not overshadow another's achievements and milestones. Families who seek respite resources, strive for flexibility, and seek creative solutions can help assure that the accomplishments of all family members are celebrated.

14. **Parents' Perspective is More Important than the Actual Disability.**

Parents would be wise to remember that the parents' interpretation of their child's disability will be a greater influence on the adaptation of their typically developing sibling than the actual disability itself. When parents seek support, information, and respite for themselves, they model resilience and healthy attitudes and behaviors for their typically-developing children.

15. **Include Siblings in the Definition of "Family."**

Many educational, health care, and social service agencies profess a desire to offer family-centered services but continue to overlook the family members who will have the longest-lasting relationship with the person who has the special needs—the sisters and brothers. When brothers and sisters receive the considerations and services they deserve, agencies can claim to offer "family-centered"—instead of "parent-centered"—services.

16. **Actively Reach Out to Brothers and Sisters.**

Parents and agency personnel should consider inviting (but not requiring) brothers and sisters to attend informational, IEP, IFSP, and transition planning meetings, and clinic visits. Siblings frequently have legitimate questions that can be answered by service providers. Brothers and sisters also have informed opinions and perspectives and can make positive contributions to the child's team.

17. **Learn More About Life as a Sibling.**

Anyone interested in families ought to be interested in siblings and their concerns. Parents and providers can learn more about "life as a sib" by facilitating a Sibshop, hosting a sibling panel, or reading books by and about brothers and sisters. Guidelines for conducting a sibling panel are available from the Sibling Support Project and in the Sibshop curriculum. Visit the Sibling Support Project's website for a bibliography of sibling-related books.

18. Create Local Programs Specifically for Brothers and Sisters.

If your community has a Parent-to-Parent Program or similar parent support effort, a fair question to ask is: why isn't there a similar effort for the brothers and sisters? Like their parents, brothers and sisters benefit from talking with others who "get it." Sibshops and other programs for preschool, school-age, teen, and adult siblings are growing in number. The Sibling Support Project, which maintains a database of over two hundred Sibshops and other sibling programs, provides training and technical assistance on how to create local programs for siblings.

19. Include Brothers and Sisters on Advisory Boards and in Policies Regarding Families.

Reserving board seats for siblings will give the board a unique, important perspective and reflect the agency's concern for the well-being of brothers and sisters. Developing policies based on the important roles played by brothers and sisters will help assure that their concerns and contributions are a part of the agency's commitment to families.

20. Fund Services for Brothers and Sisters.

No classmate in an inclusive classroom will have a greater impact on the social development of a child with a disability than brothers and sisters will. They will be their siblings' life-long "typically developing role models." As noted earlier, brothers and sisters will likely be in the lives of their siblings longer than anyone—longer than their parents and certainly longer than any service provider. For most brothers and sisters, their future and the future of their siblings with special needs are inexorably entwined. Despite this, there is little funding to support projects that will help brothers and sisters get the information, skills, and support they will need throughout their lives. Governmental agencies would be wise to invest in the family members who will take a personal interest in the well-being of people with disabilities and advocate for them when their parents no longer can. As one sister wrote: "We will become caregivers for our siblings when our parents no longer can. Anyone interested in the welfare of people with disabilities ought to be interested in us."

Chapter Seven

Remember to Breathe or You Might End Up in the ER Too: Care for the Caregiver

Feeling like my heart would beat right out of my chest, the panic had begun to set in. Looking at the triage nurse through blurred vision, I knew my situation was serious, especially when moments later I lost consciousness. Hoisting me up to the waiting gurney, the emergency room attendants quickly placed electrodes on my chest and waited for the screen to tell them what was wrong with me. "She has PVCs," they said, referring to a condition called premature ventricular contraction where the heart appears to skip a beat." The ensuing tests and cardiologist consultations led to one conclusion: a stress-related heart condition complicated by forgetting to breathe correctly.

I had done this to my body with martyr-like mentality, all in the name of getting my son well. It took two years to recover from the self-imposed damage to my health, and many more years after that to stop the next parent from doing what I did. Compromising our own health to meet the needs of our child with autism has become the quiet epidemic in our community. It isn't discussed broadly in our autism community, or even the general population, that autism parents are in trouble due to health conditions brought on by meteoric stress levels (read: *all* parents in the autism community).

It was 2003, and for all intents my life should have been coasting along. Daniel was in preschool, declared recovered from autism, and my daughter had just started kindergarten. We had been through a lot over the past few years, and no one was more grateful than me to know that the pit in my stomach over Daniel's future would one day subside. But for now it remained because the pit reminded me of my need to always be on guard when it came to his health and other needs. If I let down that guard then something would fall through the cracks. That was my unspoken battle-cry, it seemed— always be vigilant and on guard or risk the consequences. What this meant at the time was unclear, only that my anxiety was always in high gear because to do otherwise felt anathema to what I thought I had to be: vigilant.

Until I passed out in the emergency room.

Life Plans Gone Awry

Let's face it, we never checked "Autism Parent" when we listed our life ambitions. When I was in college in the eighties, autism was foreign to me. Did I even know what it was, let alone know someone with autism? Positively not. The predetermined life plan took a sharp turn. Like so many parents, I was in a sort of fog, faced with so many choices compounded by a sense of there being limited time and windows of opportunity in which to make the right decisions to help my child. The battles seemed to be constant. First, from the lack of knowledge about autism, then from the angst about what to do, and finally from the well-meaning naysayers who accompanied every decision.

As I was beginning to write this chapter, word came of another murder-suicide of an autism parent whose despair led them to do the unthinkable. Another mother who committed this heinous act said that prison was easier to handle than the "prison of autism." It made me incredibly sad to see how their lives had spun out of control. Stress became depression and then depression became relentless despair mired in grief. It took a toll on them physically, mentally, and emotionally. As autism rates escalate, there is little doubt this same scenario will continue to play out until we as a community begin to reach out and educate parents on how to help themselves on this journey before they collapse from the strain.

We are just beginning to understand how the physical toll the caregiver experiences cannot be endured without some form of negative impact. How many of them develop stress-related heart disease or autoimmune disorders? How many become dependent on medication (legal or illegal) or alcohol to cope with the anxiety? How many gain weight, lose weight, develop mental health disorders, or even life-threatening illnesses? In my own experience, this is absolutely one pitfall about autism not openly discussed enough, not commonly written about, and certainly not a huge topic of focus at autism conferences. But that will change because as our numbers increase, so too is the fallout of growing ill-health coming from the caregiver parents.

My Story

My adrenaline levels were already in high gear as we began to deal with the ongoing health issues, even before Daniel was diagnosed. Somewhere within I was screaming "Not my son!" This, in itself, was my great conflict. It was a drive like no other. The lack of information from the medical community and the tragic misinformation left me seriously disillusioned, confused, and isolated. Yet, my instinct to find the answers would drive my mind and body to levels of sustained endurance, only to have things come crashing down in every way imaginable.

As mentioned in a previous chapter, I spent many late nights on the computer doing research. That led to not getting enough sleep followed by a long day of taking my children to preschool and therapy appointments. Of course, my 2,800-square-foot home had to be immaculate for all of the therapists who would come that day (at least in my mind). Eating healthy only applied to my kids as I was "good to go" on the quickest, easiest thing I could eat over the sink. The closest semblance of exercise consisted of pushing a vacuum cleaner or running up and down the stairs with another load of laundry.

The worry I had for Daniel's future was overwhelming. I would not give in to the idea that he would not fully recover, or at least become healthier. I put extra pressure on myself to cover all of the bases; all the possible treatments would be explored. The refrigerator had twenty-five bottles of supplements, which

I had to figure out how to get into him every day. The bath had Epsom salt. The food was gluten/casein/soy free and we needed to be mindful of cross contamination. My daughter simultaneously needed attention. Sleep was elusive at times as I thought of the next treatment to consider, or Daniel woke up screaming with gastrointestinal pain.

Come the morning, I once again shifted into high gear for yet another day's battle. Most important in my mind was that sense that if I didn't do *all* that I was doing then my son would not recover—*and it would be totally my fault*. If he had a good day, everything would be okay for the moment. But a bad day meant I had failed in some way, and the angst and grief began all over again.

The price paid for this dedicated effort was my health. It began first with a shortness of breath that came and went. Then I would be lying in bed with my heart racing. I caught every cold and flu that came around and had nine sinus infections in one year. This was followed by the two trips to the emergency room in the same year with the same stress-related symptoms, including the time I passed out. I was forty years old.

One of the factors the doctors pointed out was that I simply was not breathing correctly. As I focused in on my daily duties or research I would lose sight of something as basic as needing to breathe regularly. While that may seem funny, I have to believe I am not the only one who shuts down breathing while under stress. My constant adrenaline rush meant my immune system was also in trouble as my body told me it had no more to give.

The chronic fatigue meant I needed to get a handle on my health or suffer long-term consequence. A friend of mine with a severe autoimmune condition warned me to heed the body's signals now before it was too late. Six years later, I realized how close I had come to dodging an autoimmune disorder bullet when I was diagnosed with severe adrenal fatigue, which impacted my entire endocrine system. Gratefully, I took her advice and began to reclaim my own health.

However, the path to health has a steep and multifaceted learning curve; first my son's health and then my own, which is why I speak often about developing better health habits while you still have good health and not have to carve it back. Initially,

I was at the mercy of physicians for direction and could no longer determine my own health answers as I had been doing with my son. I was prescribed medication by the cardiologist for the heart palpitations, but the medication left me incapacitated and listless, only able to lie on the couch. Since this was not going to work in the scope of being a mother, a series of other medications followed, leaving only side effects and a tremendous feeling of helplessness.

When the traditional route was a dead end, I turned to alternative practitioners and therapists. First, I went to an acupuncturist to help the adrenal glands and immune system, and to open up the diaphragm in order to breathe better. What followed were regular massages to condition my body back into relaxation and shift my ribcage from the heart (apparently caused from too much vacuuming). Easy walks in a local park followed, as well as lunches with girlfriends who were very willing to listen and remind me of the value of friendship. The late-night budget conversations had to stop and Rich would remind me to not be on the computer too late. Actually, stepping away was very difficult but necessary for the body to heal. I also began taking supplements and protein shakes, cut back on caffeine and alcohol, and tried to eat better in general.

All of these efforts paid off with an initial return to good health, though it took over a year just to feel confident in my body again. But what happened six years later is that I hit perimenopause and the early damage I had done to the body came back, only with new symptoms. This time, I had developed significant food intolerances, thyroid and hormone imbalance, and a systemic yeast overgrowth. Vested with new information from a new functional medicine practitioner, I once again began to build back my health and realized that this would now be a lifelong effort of better health habits.

Now, in my talks with other parents, the first thing I plead with them after telling my story is "Please do not let it get this bad for you." Take the time to *slow down and breathe*. Step out of the battle, game, fight, challenge, or whatever you choose to call it, in order to regroup. We are in this long term.

The best advice I got on this healing journey came from the acupuncturist who told the story of a man who had been in a

Chinese concentration camp for over a decade. He said the man had found that those who survived the camp were those who did everything they were ordered to do, but they did it S-L-O-W-E-R. So he told me to do the same. Do it, just do it slower. Don't be in a rush to get everything done all at once. So the phrase that I adopted and repeat to this day is "go slow and breathe."

At times, I wonder whether Daniel's recovery was strictly due to the determination and focus that eventually landed me in the hospital, or if he would have recovered anyway and I didn't have to let my health go through the beating I gave it. In any case, the lesson was learned. While we may not think so at the time of crisis, taking care of ourselves is definitely one thing we can control. Here are a few clues to consider when you are heading for a health crisis of your own.

You Are Headed for Health-Related Problems When . . .

- You feel isolated from family and friends
- You sleep too little or too much
- You eat sporadically or all of the time with little thought
- You catch colds and flus with regularity
- You develop stress-related conditions like heart palpitations, skin eruptions, allergies, etc.
- You develop digestion problems
- You develop autoimmune symptoms or have a flare up of a known disorder
- You reach for alcohol or medication (legal or illegal) to cope
- Your frustration level is high and your tolerance level is low
- You lose your sense of hope

The Guiltaholic in Us All

Virtually every parent on this journey is plagued by guilt, the kind that can seem crippling if we let it. In talks I have given on topics dealing with diet, IEP issues, and marriage issues, invariably there will be someone in the audience who brings up the word "guilt" or "guilty" as a way of signaling how they feel about their role and helplessness to change their situation. Guiltaholism is an epidemic in our community. It's what gets us out of bed in the morning and drives us to unsustainable levels of physical endurance, bringing with it all of the complications that any addiction brings.

At another presentation, where the audience fell into a conversation about guilt overwhelming them, I was filled with the sadness that permeates the parents in our community and determined to identify the attributes of guilt in autism parents, grandparents, and other caregivers. We are all searching for a way to forgive ourselves for our daily misgivings and our undone or neglectfully handled deeds. We seem forever mired by a form of pity for the very people we love the most. At one talk, the parents in the audience respectfully listened to each other but it was apparent they were searching for validation. More than anything, they desired a release from the guilt that now consumed their lives and reminded them of what they perceived as being their failures.

How could I reach out to them in awkward agreement, without discovering solutions to my own guilt? If I had found the answers for me to release the guilt, then why could I not offer them a definitive solution in some form? As I drove home from this presentation the answers began to roll through my mind with a sense of purpose. Remembering the anxiety in their faces, I vowed to articulate a method to begin releasing the grip of guilt in our lives. And, in turn, I would hopefully permanently release my own.

So I wrote a twelve-step program modeled after the vernacular in the twelve-step program for those with substance addiction. During the development of the program, it became obvious that the words I choose *not* to use were the very ones that seemed to cause us the most guilt. Gone from the vernacular were *do*, *don't*, *should*, and *must*. In their place came empowering thoughts that helped the guilt-ridden parent focus, encouraging them to throw away the anxieties that led to guilt. Clichés and rhetoric had to come with a sense of doable action steps, or the ideas would be tossed out. If it didn't make sense, or in any way was not realistic, then the idea was eliminated. Further, as I began writing the twelve-step program, it became apparent that the message was globally relevant. Step into the shoes of any parent and you will see that they are stepping into guilt every day in some form. It is just that some of us have come to rely on guilt's narcotic effect as our motivating force. That is when guilt's effects begin to suffocate the family.

To that end, I formed ideas that were transferable to even a parent who is dealing with everyday stresses, but yet completely applicable to those of us enduring the biggest levels of stress as the primary caregiver of a child with special needs.

Step 1 – Acknowledge that guilt is a "drug" of choice, and as such, we are in charge of the thoughts we choose to accept about ourselves.

Step 2 – Acknowledge, to ourselves and to others, that we cannot be everything. If our expectations are unreasonable then our thoughts of what is doable need to shift.

Step 3 – Acknowledge that part of our guilt is associated with our need to control all of the circumstances in our lives. We need to release ourselves from the responsibility of the demands that our desire to control brings.

Step 4 – Acknowledge that we are not responsible for the happiness of anyone but ourselves, including our immediate family members. Take full responsibility for formulating and cultivating care of you *first*.

Step 5 – Limit opportunities that can produce guilt: say no to volunteer opportunities without regret, choose friendly thoughts about yourself and others, and walk away from negative conversations that provoke anxiety about your choices.

Step 6 – Accept yourself for who you are, creating boundaries for how you will allow yourself to be treated. Release yourself from all self-imposed pretense.

Step 7 – Accept others for who they are, respecting and honoring their boundaries. Release them from any unrealistic expectations of behavior.

Step 8 – Accept that guilt is born from our fear of being perceived as inadequate, in our own eyes and those of others. Detach yourself from the fear of inadequacy.

Step 9 – Accept that guilt's only purpose is to temporarily motivate us to change direction from the path we may now be choosing. It is when guilt becomes a daily motivator that we have become addicted to its effect.

Step 10 – Accept help humbly, and without regret.

Step 11 – Listen carefully to your own inner voice of wisdom, and honor its call. It is in the whisper of our own inner voice that we understand the truth about ourselves.

Step 12 – Turn over your fears and your sense of limitations to your God, however you choose to define. As we accept a Higher Power our greater good is fulfilled. And when that happens, the paralyzing effect of guilt is permanently removed.

The Way Forward Begins with the First Step

Some of the stress triggers were easy to identify, which meant they were the first to go when the time came to reclaim my own health. First up, I found support in like-minded friends and family members, avoiding all naysayers. To this day, there is a physical reaction in me that happens when someone rhetorically says that kids with autism cannot improve or that their families cannot heal. It is tantamount to being a visceral response, and I either end up walking away or forcefully stopping the person from speaking further before re-educating them on possibilities that are unfolding in our community.

Not knowing what to do to help Daniel was my biggest stressor, and I see this same kind of stressor play out in parent after parent. Education and research, then, can be the ticket to overcoming the stress of not knowing what to do. You don't have to take my approach, but the steps to just head you and your child in the direction of finding answers is the first step in a long journey. And it is a necessary step to declaring victory over autism. If a grandparent is involved in some of the care of the child, be sure to encourage their involvement, as long as they are not opposed to you beginning the journey.

Maintaining some sort of exercise routine is essential for all of us, especially those of us susceptible to over-the-top stress levels. I found that, for me, simple yoga stretching and walking was all that I could do, which was enough for me to shed ten pounds in a few months and begin to connect with the fine art of breathing well. Other friends of mine who have children with special needs take on a more vigorous exercise regime, with one laughing that she beat back autism with every punch to the punching bag. Another friend would proclaim her workout time her total autism-free time of the day.

Eating healthy and drinking plenty of water is preached so often now that it is almost a platitude, but I submit that parents in chronic stress need to adopt healthy eating habits just as much as their children. Ideally, we move toward organic, non-processed, non-GMO, gluten/dairy/soy-free diets for our children, but we tend to fail in adopting them for ourselves because we just are not ready. At least not until our body demands we make changes. From personal experience, it is much easier to create these eating habits when you are healthy than when you are forced to due to ill health.

Supplements are another area where we can easily focus on what our children need, to the point that we forego our own needs. Supplements can add up cost wise, which is one of the reasons we choose cheaper brands if we take supplements at all. When my two older children reached puberty, they experienced a whole new anxiety level which is typical of all teens as their brains go through physiological changes. So, while I added new amino acids to their vitamin regimen, I began to look more carefully into using the same amino acids to help my growing anxiety levels associated with creeping menopause symptoms.

Not enough can be said about getting a good night's sleep. When our children were first born we were of course woken up often through the night. While I could stay home and nap if necessary, Rich had to go to work and try to function, which quickly left him with fried nerves. It is tough to tell a parent whose child wakes most of the night due to autism that they "should" get extra sleep. They know that and would love to do so, but their reality is different, and sleep eludes them. There are answers for getting a child to sleep through the night (okay, now that got your attention). I have listed "sleep help" in the resource section.

Finding healthy ways to relax can be difficult. I wish that I had figured out that meditation was a good idea long ago. If I had, I probably would not have landed in the emergency room. Others I know gravitate to hobbies, music, or counseling. It's our version of regrouping in order to carry on a little longer.

One tough area for me to accept was the need to take a break. I had to learn to say no to others' requests for my help; unless they were another autism parent (I could hardly turn down another parent). But whenever I could, I would close my eyes or read a magazine just to release from the tensions of the day. Other friends would receive respite care from outside agencies just to have a night out with their spouses or do some level of self-care. Since respite is one of those services that is not always a guarantee, it becomes all the more important to fit in moments throughout the day when you can just take a break.

As mentioned earlier, I value prayer as an effective tool to overcoming stress. When it was unclear how to help Daniel, I prayed for guidance. Even if you are not religious, there is something to be said for just turning it over to the "universe" to take over in order to give us a sense of renewal.

Finally, if possible, slow down the pace of your life. Must you be all things to all people? Or can you be content with being less to others and more available to yourself and, therefore, your family? It becomes a matter of setting priorities at some point. It also become essential to balance the demands placed on us in order to survive as the caregiver.

Burnout Is Real

During a dinner conversation with friends, I told them of my decision to step off the autism and special needs awareness stage for a while. I even said, "I want to be irrelevant." It was as though being a mentor had taken everything left in me, but I had gladly given it away with no regrets. The catalyst was when I wrote an article about care for the caregiver, which was published a year later in *The Autism Asperger's Digest*. After writing about my complete physical breakdown in 2003, it became apparent that my current schedule and activities were about to land me back in the hospital if I did not make changes.

Taking my own health for granted was something I had vowed to not do again. Yet here I was, on the cusp of taking on more than I had ever handled. At the time, I was already over committed with mentoring, speaking, and heading up a special needs support group. On top of this, I had been asked to lead a large autism group for the New England area. Oh, and did I mention I have three children with lots of activities? I had hit a wall, the proverbial "burnout" wall. Autism and all things special needs had been my life for almost eight years—from advocacy to mentoring to activism. In spite of my grandest efforts to continue to lead the charge of reaching out to the next parent, I found myself needing to pull back from it all. Over the years, I have seen the same thing in other parents who have reached a similar point in their lives.

When I made the decision to step away from it all, I knew it was for the better. But my anxiety rest mainly in the feeling that I was letting others down (again, that guilt thing). I even sought out counseling on how best to handle the potential disappointment from others over the decision to walk away. Truthfully, I might have been delusional that any of this mattered to anyone else.

Rich was especially surprised when I told him of my decision because he knew mentoring and advocacy were my sources of identity. What led up to that moment was a sincere question: "How did I get here?" How did I get to the point of sheer exhaustion and lack of joy? How did I get to where it was easy to find the fight but not the victory? When phone calls from parents became arduous, I knew something was seriously wrong. For a long time, those phone calls were my mission in life; to reach out to one more parent and give them hope. I was no longer able to do this. My family needed me in different ways and I needed to refocus attention back to a life beyond autism. It was a real crisis of identity as I begged to answer the question "Who am I anymore?"

This is another topic not widely discussed in our community. Still, it is very common to see parents in various stages of pulling back from the effort or the community as a whole. Either their child is older and they have reached a plateau on how far they believe their child would progress, or the parents are worn out from all of the effort. There is an element of guilt associated with pulling back, just from the connotation that it suggests a parent is giving up on the child, when that simply is not the case. In fact, that might have been my thinking toward other parents had it not been for the breakdown of my own motivation and resolve. Yes, my child was recovered so my battle for his health was mostly done. But there are always small battles that even the recovered families must fight. The new battle was now within me. Who was I without autism? It is something parents in our community will invariably grapple with at some point.

Finding peace with the decision to leave the special needs community for a while was difficult. But I managed to finally allow in the *acceptance* that all was well with me not being involved.

Getting Away From It All

Through the years, I have met parents who expressed a need to escape to a world without autism, even if only for a little while, in order to connect with whom they used to be before autism came into their lives.

Right before Daniel was diagnosed (although his behaviors were already overwhelming), I made the decision to "check out" for the day. I told Rich that I was going to spend a day out all by myself, all day. He felt put upon, stating that he had things to do too. But I stayed my ground and asked him if Sunday was better than Saturday because I was going one of those days. He got the message and backed off. It was a day I can still fully remember, including what I ate for lunch and how happy I felt just being alone doing mundane things. Impulsively, I bought a painting at an antique store because it evoked a feeling of happiness. It still hangs over our mantel.

Joanne* is a woman I mentored over a couple of years through a variety of autism-related events in her life. She related that one day she looked in the mirror and saw someone she didn't know any more. In two years of helping her sons with autism she had put on seventy pounds. I witnessed her heading for this breakdown and yet my gentle cautions to take care of her health didn't register until she had reached a crisis stage. She took action and lost the weight, developing new attitudes about her equal importance in the family. She would find the time in her hectic schedule to go to the gym and eat properly. She was still helping her sons, but she was now taking a more balanced approach, and found it doable to do both.

Alicia* is someone I met at a talk I was giving, and in the course of conversation I suggested she try meditating for five minutes just to clear her head before beginning her day. She finally decided to do this and found such a benefit that now she is doing longer stints of meditation regularly, along with yoga and tai chi.

Many other parents told me that their moments of respite were brief moments when they were able to watch TV or Netflix, skim through Facebook, or just relax in the bath after a long, difficult day. There was an element of guilt attached to the whole idea that they did not have the ability to find longer stretches of time in their lives to take care of themselves, because their realities were different than the average parent. A few lamented their lack of contact with their former friends who otherwise did not understand the magnitude of the stress they dealt with daily. In autism, what was once considered a small activity can become a luxury. One mother said it was the simple manicure or pedicure that allowed her to regroup.

As a mother of three daughters with autism, Kim took to marshal arts as her personal therapy. It also became a form of personal victory over her sense of helplessness. Another friend took up her magnificent artwork again, painting murals throughout the elementary school that her sons attend. A single parent relayed, "Burnout for me is very noticeable. The house is a disaster area, the child is running amuck with whatever electronic gadget keeps him out of my hair, and I'm under a blanket on the couch."

There is this false notion that parents of special needs children are "not allowed" to burn out, which sets up unreasonable expectations that can lead to exhaustion, depression, and eventually despair of endless proportions. As Terri said, "I didn't have the option to burn out; that's when I burned out. I had to get away by myself a few times, leaving the kids with hubby. The change of scenery was wonderful. During the years that leaving was impossible, I had coffee, chocolate, talking with non-autism friends, or a walk in the woods to help me out."

Some parents find it essential to be alone in order to avoid the burnout feeling, while others want to get away with their spouse to feel connected again. Amanda said, "I have to do these autism escapes alone. I don't want to deal with the effort of small talk or entertaining another person. It's just all about me, myself, and I doing what I want for me."

I have met families who recognize their child has arrived at their own plateaus, with the parents now looking to life beyond autism. Typically, these are parents of teenage children or older. They are done fighting the school system, insurance, doctors, etc. They are at a stage to just be at peace with it all. However, most parents are between stages of ebb and flow. They pour forth tremendous effort and energy, often for years, and then pull back to regroup financially, physically, mentally, and emotionally.

On the other hand, I have also seen parents who put forth minimal effort toward their child's well-being and then determine they are done. It is sad to see this because it is not necessarily *burnout* as much as it is *cop-out*. To not confuse the both, here is the difference: *burnout* occurs after a sustained period of time, energy, and concerted effort; *cop-out* is giving up with little or no effort because it is inconvenient or requires more energy than they want to expend. Some of these parents put more effort into buying electronics than they do their own child's health. Gratefully, these *cop-out* parents are clearly in the minority.

As part of this process of pulling back in order to regroup, it is important for parents to recognize there is a future for them that may have nothing to do with autism. For me, it was becoming a local newspaper reporter and writing about anything other than autism, all of which became my new identity. It was, in all frankness, what possibly saved my writing in general, so that I could once again come back and write about autism issues after I stepped away from it and gathered a new perspective.

Reconnecting to "Self" after Burnout

Once you have made the decision to step away from autism due to burnout, there is a certain settling down period where your thoughts and direction have no focus other than a need to change the current conditions. It can take up to a year for you to settle into a new mindset before you actually take the first step in a new direction. What I found helpful was taking time every day to just be quiet, letting go of the busy thoughts in order to just connect to my intuition again. I used to only be able to hear the words circulating my chaotic life. It took time to slow down enough to finally hear what my heart was telling me to do next.

Avoid time-consuming commitments while you are going through this regrouping stage. It is all too easy for a multitasking, type A personality to get sucked back into doing things for others, especially if it's something that type A person is good at. Initially, the hard part will be saying no. I had to say no to being a room parent or even chaperoning field trips. It was not the time to volunteer. It was really time to focus on healing my body and spirit. No amount of regrouping or reconnecting is going to work if your body is out of balance physically, so make the effort to rest, exercise, and eat healthy. This is the time to bring this part of your life in order if you have not done so yet.

Stay as connected to the autism community as you are comfortable. If you need a total break then do so without apology or regret. If you feel the inclination to stay in touch but need just enough of a break to feel good again, then cut back on your connections and focus on other areas of your life. You can do so while still remaining involved with your child's autism treatments and therapies.

Don't stop the *necessary* treatments or therapies. If something in your child requires your attention, then by all means look into what might be next to consider. I know many parents who step away from the autism community in order to devote themselves solely to what their child needs, as they should. In the midst of stepping away from autism, we had to look into Daniel's visual perception. It evolved into a six month vision exercise treatment plan at home, along with several trips to a doctor in New York. But I worked with Daniel on his vision exercises, incorporating the routine into my day along with meditation, exercise, and eating right.

There should be something to look forward to. You may want to plan a trip, take a college course, learn a new hobby, or just reconnect with old friends. Everyone needs to feel their life and future has a purpose. Find the ways to rediscover what that purpose is by planning something you look forward to doing. For me, I took pleasure in planning birthday parties at a homeless shelter. It was rewarding, fun, and creative, and got me to look forward to something to do every month. Some of my friends started small home businesses to provide a bit of income while allowing them to do something that got them out of the house and connecting with their broader community again.

Seek counseling and ask for help if necessary. There is no shame asking for help after burnout hits. In fact I'd like to think it should be part of the healing process in order to fully move forward. Don't follow a preconceived time frame to determine when you should be ready to start the autism battle again, if at all. You will know what you are physically, mentally, and emotionally capable of handling, and when. If your child still needs interventions and you are not ready to pick up the mantle then pass off these duties to your spouse (if this applies) until you do feel ready. It is okay to ask for help and expect it. If the other person feels hesitant to step up, do not rush to fill the void right away. They may come around to understanding their own capabilities and the need to step up in this time, when you need it most.

Checking Back In to the Battle

Checking in to start the autism battle again is not necessarily going to happen with the same level of drive and purpose as when the child is first diagnosed. It is often tempered by the parents' realization they have less to give personally. Or they know what treatment prospects are best for their child so they focus on those few, as opposed to learning about every other new therapy. They are back in gear, but are definitely down shifting their speed. For me, stepping back into autism again came in stages. First, I began to volunteer as an advocate for children whose parents were low income. I eventually got back into mentoring and some activist activities. Mostly I began to write again.

There was a time when I received a hundred emails a day, largely from autism support groups. I am now down to a handful of emails, and only a few of those have anything to do with autism.

Once I decided to step away from the community, I knew I would not be in contact with some of the most amazing people I had ever met. We only had autism in common, but we were in it together. It's a kind of bond no one ever seeks, but we wonder how we ever got by without these people in our lives.

For a while, I sat on the sidelines and applauded their continued efforts and watched some of them rise in notoriety for bringing autism awareness to the forefront. Letting go brought me back into autism from a different perspective. All of the magazine articles I have ever written, or words of wisdom passed down, have been born from personal experiences. Now, this chapter about walking away from autism is part of that same personal experience that we share in common—identity crisis and all.

If this chapter does nothing more than to allow the parent to accept their ever-changing role, to reconnect to themselves, and to once again look ahead to their own future, then this chapter has served its purpose. As much of this book has already mentioned, there is a time to heal the healer. Sometimes stepping away begins that process.

Recycling through Grief during Burnout

Julia Berle can distinctly remember she knew she was going through the grief cycle at the same time she was going through autism burnout. Her son was considered recovered from autism, but when he suddenly became ill again Julia found herself stepping back into the cycle of fear, anger, and denial, staying in denial for a period of time before she realized that her son's new symptoms needed to be addressed.

"I beat myself up a lot," she said about the delay in acknowledging her son's worsening symptoms. "We had three solid years of looking pretty damn near cured, then he started with verbal tics and ADHD."

Post-traumatic stress disorder from the autism battle lingers in the caregiver parent similar to the way PTSD lingers in the wounded soldier, bringing with it a range of emotions that can send a parent right back to the first stage of grief: fear. For Julia, her son's new symptoms meant walking down the autism path again, a path she had wanted to leave behind for a period of time in order to heal herself. When her son was diagnosed with PANDAS, Julia felt herself slide right back into the dark hole of despair.

"I felt alone again. I got very victim-y. It took me awhile to sit in it," she said with almost a sense of embarrassment because her normal persona is the antithesis of victimhood. Yet, as she wallowed in her self-pity (as she describes it), she also found within her the resolve to pull herself together for the sake of her children. "It was my unadulterated love for my children that pulled me out of it," she added.

Looking back, Julia's experience while recycling through the grief cycle and the ensuing despair gave her the impetus to go back to school, where she got her doctorate in counseling families with special needs children. She knew her experience was not unique and would give her the perspective to help the next parent move beyond their own personal grief. While it was a dark time for Julia, she boldly affirms she is now "living in Technicolor."

The Therapist's Turn . . .

Dr. Jamell White knows the signs of burnout when she sees it in her clients. As a licensed therapist in Maryland specializing in families with special needs children, she can identify the signs the moment the family walks in through the door. These signs even appear in the siblings of the children with special needs, but the primary caregiver often has to be coaxed into accepting respite help, releasing their fears and guilt over the idea that no one but them can, or is supposed to, take care of their child.

"I see the caregiver pattern," said Dr. White. "It's a never ending job and it's draining." While she encourages the caregivers to seek family and professional support, they are often overwhelmed by the entire system they have to navigate just to take care of their sick child. "And this is on top of the job of being a parent," Dr. White added. She informs them that at some point caregiver burnout is going to happen. It's a matter of time. Part of her therapy, then, is to help her clients prepare and plan for the time when they will need to rely on others to take care of their child, whether it is preparing financially or physically for their care. What she wants them to avoid is the last minute crisis where a caregiver parent falls gravely ill or waits until their senior years before making plans for the adult child with special needs.

As a therapist, she has seen the need for respite help grow in proportion to the increase in the number of children being identified with special needs, especially autism rates. But many of the families she sees either choose to wait before signing up for respite, or find the respite services are not readily available where they are located.

"I do recommend that they find additional supports for themselves, either professionals or family and friends in their lives for coordination of care," Dr. White indicates. "There is so much navigating of the system. This is added on top of the job of being a parent. It's a need for them to take a break for themselves. That need is real."

Nationwide, there is a conservative estimate that fifty million families deal with the need for respite services for their family members, including the elderly, adults with disabilities, and families of special needs children. It has long been documented that long-term respite services for primary caregivers have both monetary and physical well-being benefits for the caregiver, who often endure health complications from the strain of caring for a family member.

When state institutions were dismantled in favor of the more inclusive model of keeping children home and in their community, Congress enacted the Temporary Child Care for Children with Disabilities and Crisis Nurseries Act, which provided federal funding for respite services programs. Today, these services are administered by state agencies but paid for by both Federal and State grants because it helps reduce the cost of care if a family member is cared for at home versus by the state. States are only starting to fully address this dire need in funding for these families, often through Medicaid.

Not far from where I live is the Michael Carter Lisnow Respite Center in Hopkinton, Massachusetts, where families are able to access a variety of respite services for their children with special needs. Named after a young boy with special needs, the respite center has served hundreds of families in the area. But respite facilities like Lisnow are few in number. Friends of mine often wait months for respite care to become available, especially if their child is medically fragile and requires nursing-level respite services.

Dr. White continued by recounting that one family did not take a vacation for over thirty years while their daughter with autism lived with them. It was not until the daughter was placed in a group home that the parents decided they would take their much needed break. While Dr. White encourages creative ways for the entire family to take a vacation together, there is a need for the couples to connect and focus on their marriage. This also helps the primary caregiver to connect and reduce stress levels. Dr. White said she encourages the caregivers to take the necessary rest so as to be more available for all of their children, not just the child with special needs.

Chapter Eight

A Family's Plan of Action

Here is where the previous chapters flow into, as if this is the mouth of the river heading to the ocean. Here is where you plant the seeds for processing through grief, develop the necessary attributes of a bold parent, find your own core mantras, become savvy on the needs of your child with autism and the rest of the family, and take care of yourself if you are the primary caregiver. This is the chapter on creating your plan as a family. It is a template if you will; not etched in stone and certainly only a version of things to consider as you figure out what works for your family.

This chapter includes everything I wish I had when Daniel was first diagnosed. It is the game plan, if you will, for coping through autism and creating positive changes in the well-being of your child, as well as the family dynamics. I didn't have this plan available to me at the time, and yet my son still recovered—with a lot more anxiety and stress on us than necessary. This plan, then, is a tool to create order out of chaos, a sense of direction through the minefields, as well as to create a true feeling of confidence over the anxiety.

In formulating any kind of game plan, the first thing you create is the goal line. Where do you imagine your child (and you for that matter) ending up in say six months, a year, two years, etc.? Dream big and set the bar high on this one; if the bar is too low, then how will you know the possibilities unless you raise your expectations? In my mind, I saw the Christmas letter I would write that announced that Daniel had overcome his diagnosis of autism and was recovered. I knew it would happen. It's just that my goal was to get him there by the age of eight. Instead, it happened by the age of four. I am glad I had set a realistic goal because eight (or even older) was entirely doable for me. For the purposes of developing this first plan, create a six month goal and plan of action items that propel you into a forward momentum which will develop your bold attributes. Shooting for improved health should be one of your goals, too.

Let's say your child is older, and you have determined that your child is moving toward different needs. For you, the goal can be that your child develops self-care skills, learns to read at peer level, or develops a way to have friends. If you create the plan, the energy to execute it will surely follow, and eventually so might many of the results that you desire. If it is not everything, then at least you know that some sort of progress will be made by both the family and the child.

Now let's create a list of possible goal lines on your map to progress. Get out a sheet of paper, a book, a binder, or something that is accessible and easy to display. A huge grid sheet would be great to consider too. It has the look of a command center. Use whatever marking instrument you want. Personally, I would have used markers in various colors—highlighters, stickers, anything to create a mood of enthusiasm around the goal. At the top of the paper you can write your child's name, and the current date on the left hand side, with the GOAL and a time frame of sorts on the right hand side. Here are some samples of goals to consider:

In six months, my child will _____ (you fill in the blank).

In six months my child will: potty train, speak ten words, spontaneously play, improve stimming behaviors, etc. I probably would have put down many of these goals all into one, so I might have written "My child will blow everyone away with how far he has progressed in six months." Go for it! Put your child's picture on the goal line. You get the idea. The next road map and goal line that you create will be far more specific on the details. It will allow you to create a comprehensive plan based on your child's specific needs (age of your child is not a factor).

Next up is the specifics of how your child will get there and who will be there to help. This is the part where we create clear objectives and benchmarks (yikes, a bit of IEP talk here). I really don't like ambiguity when I am creating a plan. I like to have a checklist and to delegate some of these tasks. (Hint: it's not the primary caregiver's duty to do all of the tasks on the list.)

Here are a few ideas to illustrate this part of the plan. Put this on the same sheet of paper, or a separate one, as long as the objectives are on target with the goal. This is where you will begin to rely on your past experiences, talents, and strengths to formulate a plan. You will also potentially be calling on your current relationships to shore up for the battle that lies ahead. Every person or group involved in this process will get their own column. However, for now we will just put down the names of the parents. Start with listing the strengths of each parent and their possible connections.

Lisa	Joe
Organized	Good at negotiating
Good at finances	Understands the medical profession
Mom can help with babysitting	Company has health benefits for therapy
Good at research	Sister is a physical therapist

Therefore, the list can continue. . .

Will join a support group	Will contact physicians
Will meet with financial planner	Will attend all IEP meetings
Will ask Mom to help with childcare	Will ask sister for insight on therapy reference

Sounds like marching orders already. At least it begins to feel like organized momentum. Personally, I like deadlines for when tasks will be done, if necessary. It helps to see how the plan is moving along. Obviously, this is a hypothetical list. You will know what works best for you but it should contain some avenues not yet explored, like a different kind of resource.

Here are some questions to ask yourself as you are creating this plan and coming up with your own set of priorities.

1. What profession did you choose? Or what company do you work for? Something about this experience or connection may be a benefit to your child's health. Are you good at negotiating? Do you have a medical or nutrition background? Are you a therapist of any sort? Are you a teacher? Do you work for a company that has medical benefits? Is there another parent in your company that has a child on the spectrum as well? Have they helped you to understand steps to take? Take a moment to seek all areas of strength and opportunity in your current and past work experience. It may prove beneficial to you and your child.

2. What about your spouse? Is there something you have learned from each other that is helpful for this time in your lives? Have you saved well? What other talents do you or your spouse possess? Are you good at writing? Are you good at finances? Are you good at organizing? Are you good at internet research? Now is the time to delegate duties according to each parent's areas of strength. Is one better at the IEP process and the other better at research? If a parent is single, are there other relatives or friends who may be willing and able to assist in their areas of strength?

3. What about other relatives, friends, or neighbors? In your neighborhood, is there another parent who has a child with autism that can help you get started? Is there a support group in your area? Seek out help and information from those closest to you. If you have a friend or acquaintance in a profession of direct knowledge, now is the time to ask for guidance and help.

4. What about your child? Does your child possess unique talents or challenges that predispose you to seek out certain therapies? What are the experiences other children have with these treatments or therapies? What about your child's early years gives you an idea of what to research? How does your child relate to others? My son's relationship with his sister told me that he had the ability to emulate "normal" behavior. If you have more than one child on the spectrum, then the plan is doubled for organization purposes, with each presenting with different needs.

This can also work for single parents facing the daunting task of going it alone in the care of their child. Surround yourself with those who will help you to make and implement decisions. Make sure whatever assistance they offer uses their inherent talents, strengths, and connections. In fact, your list may already have several columns of people who are able to help you with the duties ahead. And don't be afraid to ask for any and all help where necessary.

Again, this is something I wish I had done early in the diagnosis. In spite of the fact that our son is now recovered, there were moments of more stress than necessary. This kind of delegation would have helped Rich and me to understand our individual roles in helping our son. And we might have done so with less overwhelming effort. In hindsight, here is what our list would have looked like if we had chosen to sit down and create a plan:

Daniel – January 2001	Six Month Goal: Better health evidenced by: • Better bowel movements and improved behavior • No screaming after naps! • Begins to engage more during ABA and speech sessions

Mary	Rich
Good at negotiating	Good at finances
Organized	Methodical
Time to do research	Company benefits
Mom can babysit	
Good at writing	

Therefore, the list would have continued:

Will make doctor appointments	Arrange for occasional babysitters
Will join support groups, both online and neighborhood	Will check with company benefits coordinator for service options
Will write letters to school district and doctors	Set up flex-spending medical accounts
Prepare for all IEP meetings	Set up medical checking
Implement diet changes	Will attend all IEP meetings and most doctor appointments

The tough part about this list is that you will probably be creating it at the same time you are going through the grief cycle listed in chapter 1. Having a plan provides a measure of relief, especially when facing the day-to-day anxiety of not knowing what to do to help your child or improve your family dynamics. If you are facing reluctance from your spouse or other family members about the plan you are trying to implement, then go ahead and set it up anyway, implementing the parts under your column. But also step up and ask your spouse or other relatives and friends for specific help along the way.

In our case, Rich had a tough time with the word "autism" for about a year and a half after the diagnosis. Since he was going through the grief process (stuck in the denial stage), it was incumbent upon me as the primary caregiver to push through when necessary. While I bore the burden of implementing treatments and therapies, there were times when I had to let Rich know that we needed to start a specific treatment that was going to cost a specific amount of money. He would then come out of his denial stage for a period of time and switch to what he knew how to do best, which was to ask pertinent questions and then figure out how to pay for things with careful planning.

Eventually we set up a medical credit card to pay for all our medical expenses, and to help us keep track of these expenses for tax purposes. I know that not everyone has the financial means to do this, but focusing on those things that you can do will help keep the plan in place. Believe me, we hardly could afford it ourselves, but we became creative in the process to find the necessary funds or to have insurance pay for treatments. We will go into funding resources and making a financial plan later in this chapter.

Now that the plans for delegation have been laid out, the plan can be taken to the next level. Here is what happens after the framework of your plan is established: You begin to break down the specifics of each area for each person by creating benchmarks and objectives. (I swear this is IEP talk sneaking in here.) As an example, let's take the primary goal I would have had for Daniel: *Better health, evidenced by better bowel movements and improved behavior. No screaming after naps! Begins to engage more during ABA and speech sessions.*

Instinctively, I knew that the bowel problem was part of the reason why he kept waking up from his naps screaming. If your child is in pain, crying is a way they are going to tell you. So waking up screaming after naps, mixed with the twenty or so loose dirty diapers I was changing on him, told me that they were connected. My goal was to find out what it was that was setting him off. In January 2001, I took Daniel to a Contact Reflexologist, mainly because my regular pediatrician was at a loss to offer guidance on what foods may be causing a problem for Daniel.

The Contact Reflexologist found that dairy and wheat needed to be removed from his diet. This was a huge decision because I was unsure of this type of medical modality to determine allergens, as well as my own trepidation at changing my son's diet when he seemed to gravitate to dairy and wheat foods.

But within a week of removing dairy from his diet, the screaming after his naps ceased. Whew! That goal to me was huge. There was still too much I didn't understand, so I did more research about dietary intervention for autism and found the book written by Lisa Lewis, *Special Diets for Special Kids*, which clearly outlined and explained the reasons why to do the gluten/casein-free diet. This allowed me to feel confident to move forward with dietary changes. With diet in place, Daniel's behaviors improved dramatically, allowing him to attend better during ABA and speech sessions. He was not out of the woods, but we were certainly making progress.

If this part of the plan had been written it would have looked like this:

Mary
Set up doctor's appointment to discuss bowel movement and behavior problems.

Pediatrician appointment scheduled: _____

Gastroenterologist appointment scheduled: _____

DAN doctor appointment scheduled: _____

I did not entirely understand how his bowel movements were related to his autism, so I don't think I would have initially set up a DAN doctor appointment, which is why I list the physicians in the order above. As mentioned in a previous chapter, these physicians are now certified as MAPS (Medical Academy of Pediatric Special Needs) doctors. But a physician who is well versed on treating children with autism medically is also worth considering. I recommend you speak with both your pediatrician and autism physician before either of them recommends a gastroenterologist. A GI doctor appointment typically needs a referral, and it is best to get one who is recommended by another physician. In our case, the first GI doctor, who we saw in 2001, was recommended by our pediatrician. The second GI doctor, who we went to in 2003, was recommended by our DAN doctor. There are very few who totally understand autism so the process of getting a good GI doctor may take a while.

Since Daniel's medical issues were of primary concern, they are listed at the top of our priorities. You will be doing the same by listing health issues first. Moving forward on the objective list, here is what following this list would have entailed. The line next to each category indicates whether it was completed, that a date is in place for an appointment, or a deadline established.

Contact Early Intervention agency: _____

Research behavior interventions: _____

Research possible GI problems in ASD children: _____

Purchase necessary diet change book: _____

Join online chat group with other parents: _____

Join a neighborhood support group: _____

You can plug in your specific concerns in lieu of bowel or diet issues, especially if you are dealing with a child who has seizures or other health related disorders. The list above was my portion of the duties. Rich had his own set.

Rich
Contact benefits department to discuss company's plan
provisions: _____

Set up medical checking account: _____

Set up medical credit card account: _____

Attend medical appointments when possible: _____

Speak with financial planner: _____

While it may seem as though I ended up with a longer list, the duties were actually evenly divided. Rich did his portion while still working almost sixty hours a week and commuting three hours a day. The tough part was that, because of his long hours, I often had to call him at work to relay a problem or concern that would need his involvement, if only to preempt the fact that we needed to discuss it further when he got home. That reduced the feeling of bombardment when he walked in the door. If both parents work, then the list will certainly look more equitable. But someone still has to be around to carry out the plan with the child. That is a choice that may require a third column if the daytime caregiver is someone other than the parent.

You would think that having a single plan is the end-all/be-all answer to mapping out the decisions that will lie ahead. Trust me, a plan is needed every six months in order to renew your commitment and focus on the next set of goals. As an example, when I would meet with the DAN doctor, she would ask for a new set of labs every six months to compare progress in some areas, while asking for different labs to address any new concerns that may have come up. Sitting down with her, it was clear that we had new priorities to focus on, creating a new list of goals and objectives. Likewise, as Daniel progressed in his behavior therapies, the meetings with the school district also began to change as we recognized opportunities to challenge Daniel further with amended IEPs.

This is what the next six months of planning would have looked like:

Daniel – June 2001   Goal: Better bowel movements

Get a handle on all diet concerns

Develop a comprehensive behavior plan

Add more speech services

Mary

Implement GFCFSF diet: _____

Ask support group for behavior intervention references:_____

Ask early intervention for additional speech services: _____

Have Daniel evaluated for speech concerns: _____

Because we were also dealing with Daniel's orthopedic needs, I would have added in the following objectives to help with those issues:

Set up appointment with new orthopedic specialist:

_____

Work with physical therapist to help Daniel's low muscle tone:

_____

Add in some occupational therapy sessions through early intervention: _____

One other thing I would have added to this list would have been embrace the education process, meaning my education about all things autism. With six months and counting since developing a plan, the real priority would be to attend some sort of autism conference that would spell out the various treatment and therapy options available. You can certainly consider this in the first six months, but for sure by the second six months. Since information changes regularly, what was once "alternative" may now be mainstream. Therefore, by the sixth month you should be planning to attend an autism conference in your area or out of state. Some states even offer reimbursement for parents to attend these conferences. It is worth asking your contact at your Early Intervention or state agency if this is available or if there are any private organizations that fund these requests from parents.

Attend autism conference in October: _____
Attend behavior conference in Anaheim next March:

_____

Ask online and local support groups for treatment considerations: _____
Research potential treatment options and discuss with MAPS doctor: _____
Or you may want to research potential MAPS doctors online if you do not have one.

It is not a bad idea to develop a simultaneous or separate goal sheet for educational goals and objectives, even though the IEP should be all encompassing. This is not to say you need to recopy the IEP to your own sheet at home, but it is to say that your role in the IEP, including understanding the IEP process, needs to be placed on a goal sheet at home.

Recall my story of how I was in "coast" mode, meaning I sort of just let the district tell me how things worked and how I was supposed to go along with everyone up to the point of signing the IEP. Gratefully, I turned this perspective around before the first IEP meeting came. However, if I had this plan in place then, this is how it would have looked:

Daniel: May 2002   Goal: Develop a comprehensive IEP with the district that includes 1:1 speech, preschool services, ABA at home and in school, physical therapy, and occupational therapy.

Purchase a book about the IEP process: _____
(I already mentioned that I like *The Complete IEP Guide* by Lawrence Siegel, mainly because it has some terrific letter samples to consider using as it pertains to your child.)
Begin writing letters to the school district: _____
Set up appointment with outside speech pathologist: _____
Ask private preschool administrator to attend IEP meeting:
_____
Notify school district of the intent to record the IEP meeting:
_____
Meet with every member of the IEP team in advance of meeting: _____
_____ - Speech pathologist
_____ - Psychologist
_____ - Sped director
_____ - Occupational therapist
_____ - Physical therapist
_____ - Behavior therapist or coordinator of behavior programs

---

Up next is the value of organizing this whole process of scheduling appointments, reading literature, and attending conferences. While it may seem daunting to put together all of this in writing (especially when our day-to-day lives cause us to fly by the seat of our pants), it is the process of writing down the goals and objectives that will lead to a real sense of confidence and organization.

How do you discern that the complexities of this process are actually benefiting your child? First, *you* feel empowered by the degree of organization in this plan, enough to be able to make decisions, which alone will help your child. What we did was to create a system that allowed us to have conversations with all physicians and therapists based on the careful diary I had created that outlined Daniel's medical history. It illustrated the treatments and medical appointments we had sought, as well as the result from everything we had tried. This was me creating data and a means to monitor the progress of the decisions. Under the category of organization, the plan would look like this (and this can fall into the category of either parent):

Create a continuous running diary of medical appointments:

_____

Create a continuous running diary of therapy appointments:

_____

You may combine these two diaries into one, but your physicians may be more interested in the medical component of your child's history. You will want to place all important documents in a readily accessible binder that you will be taking with you to various appointments. You can have them in a hanging file at home too, but definitely they will need to be in an organized binder to be the most effective.

Place all reports from physicians into a binder (divide by physician): _____

Place all lab reports into the same medical binder:

_____

> Place all therapists reports into a binder (divide by therapist):
>
> _____
>
> Place all IEPs and data progress sheets into a binder (divide by service category): _____

At times, I would bring multiple binders to physician's appointments, depending on the concerns we had about Daniel at that time. At the IEP meetings, I had a full binder with Daniel's name on the front, indicating to the team that I was on top of Daniel's progress. Often, I would refer to a data sheet, a report, or something they had sent me to form a conversation in the IEP meeting. It allowed us to focus in on Daniel's specific needs, eventually allowing him to progress enough to reduce his need of services.

Moving back to the command center plan still in play, our next action plan, which would be the third plan we have created, would have looked similar to this:

> Daniel: January 2002   Goal: A better immune system for Daniel; make progress with ABA program; learn to speak; better bowel movements (always on my list).
>
> Begin IVIG infusions: _____
> Add probiotics to supplement regimen: _____
> Adjust vitamin/mineral regime where necessary: _____
>   Cod liver oil_____
>   Cobalt mineral: _____
>   Calcium/magnesium: _____
> Add more speech to IEP: _____
> Run new set of labs to determine IgG food intolerances:
>
> _____
>
> Attend local parent group meetings: _____

You will notice that I did not put my name under a delegation list. At this point, my routine is under control and we know specifically who is doing what. Although there are still times when we need to call in reinforcements (a.k.a. Grandma) to handle some babysitting needs.

The in-home program should also have its own set of discernible goals. Yes, most of us have services through the school districts, but it is still important to have your own programs in and out of the home. In our case, the school district provided an in-home behavior therapy program, as well as one at the school. But we supplemented what the district could not provide in his overall IEP to ensure that progress was made in all areas. For instance, we added in additional physical and occupational therapy to address Daniel's overall development, not just academic benchmarks. Progress notes were added to the binder, but to plan for these therapies would have looked like this:

Daniel: June 2002   Goal: Better muscle tone and core strengthening; learn to swim; less sensitivity to noise.

Look into gymnastics program with occupation therapist:
_____

Check on insurance paying for PT/gymnastics program:
_____

Look into local horseback riding program: _____
Check on insurance paying for horseback riding program:
_____

Look into sound therapy: _____
Ask school district to add in a sound-based program: _____
Check on insurance paying for outside sound therapy:
_____

You are getting the picture that your command center is all encompassing yet flexible enough to meet your needs. Having it right there in front of you keeps you focused on the goals and aware of the progress being made toward those goals. If you want to add to the goal plan as you get going, do so with realistic expectations for you and your child. You alone know what you can afford in time, energy, and money.

Speaking of money, here is how to zero in on the financial component of treating autism. Unfortunately, there is no one way to finance autism at this time except that some states are moving to mandate some behavior therapies into insurance plans. Insurance companies are remiss to accept autism biomedical treatments of any sort, declaring any and all treatments and therapies to be "experimental." That is why most biomedical treatments are coded with anything other than autism related. No worry, there are ways around everything, or at least most everything that has a price tag on your child's well-being.

Creating a financial plan to help your family through the autism journey is very much like your own financial plan for your typical family's future. In fact, it might not be a bad idea to sit down with your financial planner or accountant to discuss alternative means for creating a cash flow during periods when the money may be the most needed, and the tightest. For Rich and me, this decision was simply made by contacting our local financial planner to discuss taking loans out on our investments, then placing a phone call to our accountant to figure out ways to plan for recouping some of these expenses in our tax return.

Following this conundrum about how to pay for things, we seriously looked at our spending habits in all things not related to our family's needs. Money was a constant concern for us as the needs often outweighed the income. For my part, I was struggling to maintain a sense of normalcy, and a sense of sanity, during the whole autism journey. At times, that meant taking my children on excursions or out to lunch, which of course added to the monthly total expense. For Rich's part, he initially had a hard time accepting that gluten/casein-free foods really do cost a bit more, although they have become cheaper and more plentiful since the early days of starting this diet. But Rich and I were mostly united in the common goal of doing whatever we needed to help Daniel return to health.

Families who must deal with long-term care planning for their child with special needs are the ones who will benefit the most from careful planning. This will also go a long way to lessening the fear and stress of wondering how your child will be cared for in their adult years. When it came time to set up our family's living trust and dependent-care proxy if anything were to ever happen to either Rich or me, we sat down with a lawyer to discuss our wishes and to map out how Daniel and Theresa would be cared for long-term should the need arise. We chose guardians for them, included careful instructions on how Daniel was to be cared for, and detailed how the assets would be used toward the care of both. It was difficult to have this kind of conversation, but it was necessary to ensure our children were protected.

Unfortunately, I have met a handful of parents over the years who were much more interested in their status-symbol expenditures than the care of their child's medical issues. It would astound me to speak to parents who would declare that they couldn't implement a gluten/casein-free diet because it was too expensive, but then in the same breath discuss the new plasma screen TV they had just purchased or the vacation home they were building. It didn't add up. It was a matter of priorities for sure.

Getting back to the financial plan, let's start with the obvious areas: what does my child need over the next six months? (Add in twelve and eighteen months for future expenses too.) Calculate the potential costs and whether or not it can be covered by a flex spending account, a medical checking account, insurance, or by other means. Flex spending through your employer can also be used for child care if you have an outside provider that you initially pay for out of pocket.

Flex spending account: $2500 total
Cost of supplements: _____
      Cod liver oil: $20 x 6 = $120
      Liquid multivitamin: $50 x 3 = $150
      Mini minerals: $100 x 6 = $600

List any current medication expense and pad the amount for some that are unforeseen, including those for your other children, you, or your spouse.

Medical checking account: $1000/6 mo.
Cost of medications: list planned totals
    Depakote: $20 co-pay insurance
    Gastrochrom: $400 month, no insurance
    Flagyl: $20 co-pay insurance
    Nystatin: $20 co-pay insurance
    Benedryl: $10 paid for by flex spending account
    Other medications: $20 paid for by flex spending account

Next up, we list potential costs for therapies and treatments.

Possible loan, flex spending, and insurance coverage:
                      $_____
Cost of biomedical treatments: _____
    Cranial sacral: $40 co-pay insurance
    Autism doctor: $400 for office visit medical checking
    Chelation therapy: $100 x 6 flex spending or insurance
    (depending on what is covered)
    Lab reports: $300 co-pay Insurance
    Hyperbaric oxygen sessions: $2,000, starting in six months
    ($200 x 10) – possible payment through asset loan.
    Physical therapy: $20 co-pay insurance, plus school services
    Outside speech: $100 per session, insurance, flex spending
    and asset loan

What is not included in this planning process is the cost of gluten/casein/soy-free foods. Your current food budget and whether or not you make your GFCFSF foods from scratch (or use another dietary plan) will determine the overall cost of your food bill. If I were to give a conservative answer, my estimate is that the cost of your food may go up a third (again, just a guess based on my own experiences). There are ways to cut down on the food bill, such as making foods from scratch and joining local food co-ops that share in the purchase of large bulk items. What you spend in food, however, is mitigated by the change in the behavior of your child and the overall improvement of your family's diet. You will notice a decrease in the amount of processed foods that are purchased, including those that contain additives and preservatives, thus lessening the health-related issues that arise from these unnecessary ingredients.

If, for budgeting purposes, your plan needs to include a more comprehensive list of specialty foods, then that can be a part of a separate list. Such a list can also be used during tax season to show that you have a higher food bill due to medical needs. Speak with your accountant on how this can be turned into a tax write-off. Just remember that you will need to keep receipts. By keeping copious records, you can find ways to off-set the financial impact of autism. It will still be an adjustment of major proportions, but with a plan in place the priorities are made clear.

If you are a low income family, this is all feasible for you as well. One woman I spoke with was able to provide a gluten/casein/soy-free diet to her two children with autism by using food stamps. Oh, and I should mention that she also was able to get Medicaid to pay for some of the autism treatments for her children. (I know, it was a miracle.) Lesson to us all: a determined parent trumps bureaucratic obstacles every time.

Let's not forget the cost of educational advocacy. It is my hope that parents will feel confident enough to be their child's advocate in all areas, including the educational setting. But for many, there is a need to hire advocates and/or special education attorneys. Other parents may simply be too overwhelmed or emotionally connected to their child's educational needs to be objective during the IEP process. The special education attorney or advocate can help facilitate an outcome that is more in line with the child's educational needs than if the parent lobbied on their own.

Cost of advocate: $2000 paid for by asset loan or by local state agency.

Cost of outside psychologist evaluation: $4000, paid for by asset loan or by school district.

Cost of medical evaluation: $20 co-pay insurance

Cost of outside speech pathologist: $500, paid for out of pocket or loan

As you can see from the above example of costs, the price of an advocate can run into the thousands of dollars. Attorneys are certain to be even more, which is why I highly recommend parents getting good at the IEP process. If you become educated and assured in IEP issues, then you become a strong advocate for your child throughout the year, not just during the once-a-year IEP meeting. In addition, you will save thousands of dollars in legal expenses, money that can be better spent on getting your child well. This is one area where I excelled. Go figure how my background in retail fully prepared me to be my son's advocate. As a result of not having to spend money on attorneys or advocates, our funds were freed up to do outside therapies that helped Daniel tremendously.

Final Tips

1. Create a six month plan complete with doable goals, objectives, and benchmarks for your child, as well as anything that pertains to the rest of the family.

2. Outline the strengths of each parent and anyone else connected to your child's well-being. Notate connections to anyone or anything that may be of help to your family.

3. Once you have identified the areas of strength, as well as the areas of connections, then create a list under each person or "connection," complete with duties outlines and a line to indicate a task has been accomplished or an appointment date has been secured.

4. As you create this framework of the plan, you will be filling in details as you head into the next six months, even areas that are to be addressed in following plans. Let me be clear: this plan is flexible and available for change as the need arises. It is absolutely worth the effort as it creates the way to become both organized and self-assured. You develop your own road map for your child without waiting for others to tell you what is important. You know because the plan is in front of you, prominently reminding you of your role in the quest to help your child.

5. As the plan progresses and you begin to see the wide open space of possibility ahead, then begin to create a more challenging plan. As your child progresses—and they most certainly will—you can then turn your attention to the next areas of concern; sort of like speeding up the map objectives. As an example, we planned to look into chelation as a form of treatment to reduce the level of heavy metal toxicity. But because Daniel's yeast levels were consistently too high, we kept pushing off chelation until such time that the coast was clear on the yeast. As luck would have it, the IVIG treatments we did for Daniel had a chelating effect, thus eliminating the need to consider a separate chelation therapy. Likewise, you will be faced with opportunities to add something to your child's regimen because a treatment became available, the timing was right, or your child's needs changed, warranting a shift in focus on the plan. This is also part of keeping the plan flexible and workable.

6. Next up is the part of the plan that concentrates on other family members. The primary caregiver must have a plan for respite, both in time and focus. If stress levels are at a constant high, then the primary caregiver will burn out too quickly. This part of the plan should include time to do private matters, to exercise, even to go out with a friend. It does not include housework as part of the caregiver's "private" time. Under this section may be items like haircut appointments, a scheduled physical, and even date nights. It's a long journey, and everyone must be put into the plan of action.

7. If necessary, add action items for other family members. This way, as you navigate the intricacies of your child's autism, you are equally connected to the needs of the other children. This may sound arduous to continue to put day-to-day issues on the planning board, but in the end it is all about surviving autism with the family dynamic intact.

8. As mentioned above, there needs to be a separate action plan for academic concerns. Yes, you have your standard

IEPs, but what about everything else that goes into academic progress? Do you have any private therapists, or do you want to see if there are ways to get therapy paid for through insurance or state agency funds? The point is that, because this section can eventually end up looking like a company reorganization chart, it is wise to have a separate action plan for just academic pursuits. If you feel better having the plans in one area, then continue to combine them. Over time, you may find ways to separate various components of the plan into more specific areas. But to get started, keep it simple and useable.

9. Purchase any and all necessary supplies to create a plan that is easy to navigate visually, as well as a method to organize your efforts. These two steps will keep you on track as your child continues to improve.

10. Under the plan, be sure to include a section about supplements your child is currently taking, including dosages. Part of having the plan is that you can see what works for your child, which also gives you an idea if something is causing side effects. In autism, it is best to have regular "vitamin vacations" and come off of all supplements (except probiotics and digestive enzymes) in order to determine if the supplements have become toxic in any way. The idea is that as you reintroduce a supplement after a week or two, the body will then react adversely if a supplement has become toxic or harmful in any way. So, a "vitamin vacation" needs to be listed on the plan at least twice a year. Ask your child's physician for guidance on this schedule if you feel uneasy about any part.

The bottom line is that by the virtue of having a plan you are now firmly in control of what lays ahead. With a plan of action you can see where future expenses may occur, as well as the progress you anticipate happening with your child. With a plan, you can see where time for other family members is doable and necessary in order to create a cohesive balance in the family dynamic. Also, with a plan, the overwhelming sense of "what do we do?" seems to lessen right away and in its place a new "take-charge" mentality is born.

Navigating this journey with a plan in place means that we have declared victory over the impact of autism on our family. It is the start toward better days, better health, and well-being for everyone.

Chapter Nine

Recovery is Achievable!
Obliterating the Myths of Autism

Our family's victory over autism is not unique. There are literally thousands of families who believe their child improved significantly or overcame autism entirely. How this was achieved differs for each child. But the one thing they *all* had in common was at least one proactive parent to lead the way. None of these families found recovery, or improvement, in the same manner or method, but embraced a wide breadth of ideas until they found the keys to success for their child. They were diligent, profusely inquisitive, and bold in their decision making. None were reticent to ask questions, and all enjoyed a sense of disdain for conventional methods of treating autism.

Recovery versus Cured

What needs to be said here is that **recovery is not the same thing as cured**. In fact, those of us who have a child who is considered to be recovered from autism don't use the word "cure." It simply is not an accurate description. Cure implies you are forever done with whatever ailment you at one time had. Think "cured of cancer" or another malady that is truly curable. For autism, the word recovery is more appropriate because it connotes the idea that, while the child no longer has autism symptoms, the underlying biological predisposition of the autism is always present (immune system, gastrointestinal, neurological issues).

Most of us continue to build back our child's health even after they no longer qualify for the autism diagnosis. In our case, Daniel was determined to be indistinguishable from a typical four-year-old and displayed no overt autism symptoms, when at one time he was fully affected. Even after that proclamation by his pediatrician, we still had not gotten a handle on his chronic diarrhea, so we scheduled an appointment with the gastroenterologist in New York for a full endoscopy/colonoscopy. The result was that Daniel's gut still had issues, which prescription medication remedied within two weeks.

While he went from twenty-seven hours a week of school services down to two hours for just speech as he entered kindergarten, he was now showing signs of having auditory processing delay which caused him to not process sound—or verbal teaching instructions—correctly. We then modified his IEP to further accommodate him in the classroom. We also took him for sound therapy, with the end result being that his cognitive skills increased, making him one of the top students in his first grade class.

By second grade, we noticed he was having a hard time physically keeping up on the soccer field, which ended up with additional physical therapy, followed by hippotherapy (physical therapy on a horse) to strengthen his core muscles. By third grade, we noticed he had vision perception problems, which eventually led to him getting prism lenses and vision therapy. All of it paid off with improvements to his health and abilities. He did well enough in school but was challenged in executive functioning and organization skills, but, then again, so were the typical children in his age group.

By the time he was in middle school, he no longer needed an IEP and was put on a 504 accommodation plan instead. In high school, he continued to make strides but there was still quite a bit of encouragement needed to get him involved with school activities, not unlike many kids his age. His impulsive nature led to him wanting to run everywhere he went, which he eventually dialed back. Still, we had a typical child in so many ways and each milestone was celebrated. He joined the pep band, and when he showed up at his first football game in his band uniform I nearly cried with joy. It was an overwhelming emotion of gratitude for a moment that, at one time, I feared would never happen for him. Of course, I took loads of pictures, which completely embarrassed him. But I didn't care because I was going to capture this moment.

Even when he was grounded for behavior that many teens do, there was a part of me that was grateful I was a mom that got to do so. Absurd to some, but for those who worry for their child's future, I bequeath to you the opportunity to one day ground your child for doing something they should not have done.

A funny anecdote was when Daniel went off to a dance at the school, and I told him that two of the chaperones were friends of mine and they would be keeping an eye on him. It was a lie, but the outcome was that he "behaved" well enough to be bored at the dance. We laughed when I told him it was a ruse to make him wonder which one was "watching" him. The typical aspect part of all of this made me wish that every parent had this opportunity with their child too. Grounding your teen is a milestone and one we need to hope for one day. Well, as long as it doesn't come with a call for bail money, at least.

Recovery Stories Are Everywhere

There are so many stories of kids who are recovering or improving from autism that it would literally take volumes of books to list them all. Really. Since reading Karyn Seroussi's account of her son's recovery back when we first began this journey, there have been a number of books written detailing children recovering from autism. Three more books were published while I was writing this one, and I knew of two others that were in the works. The word is spreading that what was once thought impossible is now achievable.

In January 2013, the US National Institute of Mental Health (NIMH) concurred:

> Some children who are accurately diagnosed in early childhood with autism lose the symptoms and the diagnosis as they grow older, a study supported by the National Institutes of Health has confirmed. The research team made the finding by carefully documenting a prior diagnosis of autism

in a small group of school-age children and young adults with no current symptoms of the disorder.

The report is the first of a series that will probe more deeply into the nature of the change in these children's status. Having been diagnosed at one time with an autism spectrum disorder (ASD), these young people now appear to be on par with typically developing peers. The study team is continuing to analyze data on changes in brain function in these children and whether they have subtle residual social deficits. The team is also reviewing records on the types of interventions the children received, and to what extent they may have played a role in the transition.

"Although the diagnosis of autism is not usually lost over time, the findings suggest that there is a very wide range of possible outcomes," said NIMH Director Thomas R. Insel, MD "For an individual child, the outcome may be knowable only with time and after some years of intervention. Subsequent reports from this study should tell us more about the nature of autism and the role of therapy and other factors in the long term outcome for these children."

The study, led by Deborah Fein, PhD, at the University of Connecticut, Storrs, recruited 34 optimal outcome children, who had received a diagnosis of autism in early life and were now reportedly functioning no differently than their mainstream peers. For comparison, the 34 children were matched by age, sex, and nonverbal IQ with 44 children with high-functioning autism, and 34 typically developing peers. Participants ranged in age from 8 to 21 years old.

Prior studies had examined the possibility of a loss of diagnosis, but questions remained regarding the accuracy of the initial diagnosis, and whether children who ultimately appeared similar to their mainstream peers initially had a relatively mild form of autism. In this study, early diagnostic reports by clinicians with expertise in autism diagnosis were reviewed by the investigators. As a second step to ensure accuracy, a diagnostic expert, without knowledge of the child's current status, reviewed reports in which the earlier diagnosis had been deleted. The results suggested that children in the optimal outcome group had milder social deficits than the high functioning autism group in early childhood, but had other symptoms, related to communication and repetitive behavior, that were as severe as in the latter group.

The investigators evaluated the current status of the children using standard cognitive and observational tests and parent questionnaires. The optimal outcome children had to be in regular education classrooms with no special education services aimed at autism. They now showed no signs of problems with language, face recognition, communication, and social interaction.

This study cannot provide information on what percentage of children diagnosed with ASD might eventually lose the symptoms. Study investigators have collected a variety of information on the children, including structural and functional brain imaging data, psychiatric outcomes, and information on the therapies that the children received. Analysis of those data, which will be reported in subsequent papers, may shed light on questions such as whether the changes in diagnosis resulted from a normalizing of brain function, or if these children's brains were able to compensate for autism-related difficulties. The verbal IQs of the optimal outcome children were slightly higher than those with high functioning autism. Additional study may reveal whether IQ may have been a factor in the transition they made.

"All children with ASD are capable of making progress with intensive therapy, but with our current state of knowledge most do not achieve the kind of optimal outcome that we are studying," said Dr. Fein. "Our hope is that further research will help us better understand the mechanisms of change so that each child can have the best possible life."[1]

---

[1] National Institute of Mental Health, "Small Group with Confirmed Autism Now on Par with Mainstream Peers - NIH-Funded Study," press release, January 15, 2013, http://www.nimh.nih.gov/news/science-news/2013/study-documents-that-some-children-lose-autism-diagnosis.shtml.

While many of us in the community embraced that recovery was finally acknowledged as possible, the study also left open for interpretation the idea that the children just "outgrew" autism or were not diagnosed properly to begin with. Daniel was an original candidate for this study, which meant that I had the opportunity to speak to the researchers who conducted it. Of specific concern to them was that the child's behaviors were clearly delineated in all reports as symptomatic of autism, meaning there had to be more than a neurologist's diagnosis for the researchers to accept the report into the study. The child's behaviors had to lead to the conclusions and needed to be in the written report.

In Daniel's case, there were two individual diagnoses from separate neurologists, but neither of them included enough details about his behaviors in their report. There was the early intervention report which did detail his behaviors, but there was no diagnosis of autism, only PDD-NOS. The researchers insisted the diagnosis had to say "autism," not just PDD-NOS, in order to qualify for the study. There were three school district psychologists who labeled him with autism, along with his behavioral testing scores, but this still was not enough for the researchers.

In a conversation about the volumes of material provided to lead researcher Dr. David Black, he asked to have access to Daniel's pediatric records to comb through and find the elements that "proved" he displayed symptoms of autism. By this time, I was no longer interested in participating in the study. It was as if I was once again defending the idea that Daniel's path to hell and back was a sheer "misdiagnosis," which is the only reason he could actually recover. In another conversation with Dr. Black, I told him all the steps we took to get Daniel well, from diet to IVIG to behavior therapies. He told me that another child in the study had also recovered with the help of IVIG therapy. I cautioned him to not put too much stock in any particular treatment modality since every child was different in how they responded. I did tell him, however, that the one thing the children in the study had in common was a proactive parent leading their own research treatment study, with the lab being their home and the subject their child. He laughed and said that I might be right.

It must have been another disorder, not autism. That has been thrown at me and others who dare say we have a child recovered from autism. It comes mainly from within our own community, oddly enough. It's as if we are anathema to the whole thought of what autism is supposed to be, and we are upsetting the status quo that wants to *accept* autism and not change our children. They fail to mention that we don't want to change our children, just make them healthier. Recovery, then, is a return to health and well-being. If our children are still quirky, we could care less. But we want them to be able to navigate society in some way, and not be in pain.

I was asked to speak at a conference that featured educators from throughout the New England area. The conference organizer contacted me because of my advocacy with families in the area, and she asked me to speak on what educators need to know about autism. When I mentioned to the organizer that my son was recovered from autism, she took a deep breath and paused a bit, before finally saying, "Well, there has to be room at the table for diverse opinions." I took this as a signal that she disapproved of the whole thought that children with autism should even be treated, and that children ought to be left alone. If it was just a quirky child, there would be no battle. But we are dealing with very sick children who exhibit a host of comorbidities and are at risk for harm due to wandering, seizures, immune system dysfunction, abuse, neglect, and self-injurious behaviors. Who would not want to treat a child who clearly needed medical help? And if the child did need help, why must it always be a pharmaceutical remedy? That, then, is the challenge in this book. The answers are out there. It is up to you as the parents and caregivers to find them.

Just Getting Started Is Half the Victory over Autism

Step into the autism battle and you will see you are surrounded by those who are declaring victory over autism and the impact it has on their families. You meet parents who are simultaneously tenacious, audacious, inquisitive, intuitive, optimistic, assertive, and fearless.

My friend Erin Griffin said, "But Mary, not every child is going to do well on the DAN protocol or a diet. I've met those parents who have done everything, and nothing they tried had worked for their child."

"True," I said, "but at least they got started."

Erin had to agree. In her case, the DAN protocol and GFCF diet wasn't enough for her sons. Eventually, a friend suggested she look into the Yasko protocol, which was developed by Dr. Amy Yasko. It took a different approach than the DAN model, but still built on the principle of finding what works for the individual child. Because of how well her own sons had done on the treatments, Erin now speaks about the Yasko protocol and moderates the Yasko discussion board. If she had not at least started down the path of discovery through her initial step, she never would have found Yasko or any other answer that would have helped her sons. I liken it to "pulling a thread" with the idea that once you start you will be led to finding the answers by virtue of taking the first step, which invariably leads to another one, and so on.

For Erin, she found that her sons presented so differently that a universal method for treating them both was not working. When she decided to try the Yasko protocol, the boys were evaluated for their individual genetics to determine what type of treatment they would benefit from most. That was when they both began to improve. She believes that had she not implemented the treatments recommended in the Yasko protocol for them, then they would be in restrictive group homes needing high levels of care. Instead, they are now happy young adults working on independent-living skills.

Mary Beth Palo found that her son did not respond to standard ABA behavior therapy. But when he began to imitate scenes he saw on video, the idea stuck for her to begin videotaping "typical" behavior in order for him to learn in a way that he could connect. The video modeling she developed for her son amazed his ABA therapists, crediting the therapy for all of her son's skill achievements.

Mentoring her over the phone and email (she still refers to me as that crazy lady in California), Mary Beth implemented diet and DAN protocol, but they had their own shortcomings too. She still, however, credits diet and other treatments with healing her son's weakened immune system. Because she had started down the path of discovering what worked for her son, she attended an autism conference where she met a doctor who later would discover a malformation on her son's brain known as the Chiari 1 malformation, which was the possible cause of his seizures and would require surgery to correct.

When she visited the first neurosurgeon to discuss options, he told her that yes, her son had a Chiari 1, but he would not do surgery because surgery was not a "cure" for autism. Mary Beth was astounded. She had gone there to seek medical advice for the Chiari 1, not a magical cure for autism. The worst part of this is that he is not the only physician to refuse treatment of a child with autism, believing the parents are seeking to "cure" autism rather than simply correcting a serious medical condition.

Two weeks later, she came in contact with another neurosurgeon at a leading New York hospital who agreed to do the surgery. Six weeks after surgery, her son's seizures stopped and the language was flowing. However, the neurosurgeon credited the video modeling as being the precursor to her son regaining his speech pattern. As the doctor explained, the video modeling helped form the neurons in the brain that would one day produce a speech pattern. The surgery removed the final barrier to finding his speech.

When Mary Beth recognized that other children with autism could learn from video modeling like her son, she continued to expand the concept into a company called Watch Me Learn, which began to be used by school districts throughout the country. One day, I happened to call Mary Beth just as she was heading out the door for a diving lesson for her son. "What kind of diving," I asked. "Scuba?" She explained how he had taken up springboard diving after watching Greg Louganis videos over and over. At the time, he was fast becoming a champion springboard diver, with several TV news outlets running features on his story. Of course, I could only shout into the phone with excitement, especially knowing the ups and downs of their journey. So, while the standard treatments did not work for her son, Mary Beth figured out what did just by getting started.

Recovery Is Just the Beginning

In the early days of seeking answers, when I sat in Lisa Ackerman's living room with the other autism parents, I met Christina Adams, a local Orange County mother with a son a couple of years older than Daniel. Fast forward five years, and we connected at an autism conference where we had margaritas to toast the recovery of our sons. We were both at the conference as speakers, with Christina speaking about her new book, *A Real Boy*, chronicling her son's climb out of autism. In that toast, we acknowledged the achievement of recovery while also recognizing that we would never be done with autism. It's an odd realization when you understand that losing the diagnosis of autism is just the beginning. I often wonder what "done" looks like. For me, I decided done might be when Daniel graduates college and buys me dinner. Maybe then I will begin the release of autism to a time of "used to be."

Some parents are reluctant to acknowledge that their child had autism at one time, with several parents I know going to the extent of sealing both medical and school records to protect this information from ever being known. It was naïve of me to think that the stigma of "recovering from autism" would one day not exist, a belief that led me to use my son's name in articles, while other parents were using pseudonyms. Other friends of mine lament the fact they didn't change their child's name in articles they wrote about him or her. It isn't that they are ashamed, only that their child is potentially left to explain the "recovered" part of his journey to prospective employers. It is one of those things I wondered too. Would it be a game changer in the work world if a potential employer knew that he at one time had autism? My hope is that the stigma and discrimination about autism will cease to be an issue at all.

Girls Recover Too!

According to the latest statistics, boys are five times as likely to be diagnosed with autism as girls. However, the number of girls being diagnosed with autism has been increasing steadily. There is a prevailing belief that girls are often more severe than the boys. Theories have ranged from genetic combinations to the effect that hormones play. It has been theorized that testosterone plays a role in why boys are more susceptible than girls, but that estrogen has a greater impact on the health, behaviors, and symptoms of girls diagnosed with autism.

When Daniel was receiving his IVIG, he was often scheduled at the same time as another girl who was a year older than him, and presented with significant immune system and cognitive challenges. The mother and I became friendly, exchanging emails and phone calls. By the time the girl was five years old, she no longer could be diagnosed with autism and entered the classroom, needing no further support except for speech services. It is always with a measure of trepidation that a parent talks about the momentous occasion of their child entering a regular classroom, hoping that the child can fit in with their peers and succeed in the classroom. But the girl's progress in the classroom and milestone success proved this was no mistake. She indeed had recovered too.

Not long ago, I attended an autism conference where children who had recovered were asked to come speak (no, Daniel was not one of them). One girl took us all by surprise as she eloquently spoke about once having non-verbal autism, and how she was functioning fine today. It was her choice of words, ending with the statement, "Don't give up," that prompted the parents to give a standing ovation. My own observation is that girls and boys differ little in their severity and are equally likely to recover or improve.

Connection to the Autism Family Community Is Crucial!

In the early days of discovering answers for Daniel, I was on a bunch of Yahoo autism groups, which was the preferred communication method before Facebook took over. Those groups were like a connection to the outer world of autism families, especially important since we can feel so isolated in spite of our proximity to other autism families in our community. We needed the seeming anonymity of the internet, where our questions were answered and our frustrations expressed. The online community is where I first came in contact with autism lingo, new treatments, and therapies and doctors to consider. It was also where I began to meet people who would eventually become my friends, even if we never met face to face. In fact, I met virtually all of my mentees online before I ever spoke to them on the phone or in person.

One of these online friends is Amanda, a single mother with a beautiful daughter she calls Peach*. I first came in contact with Amanda through email when she contacted me after reading the story about Daniel's recovery, asking questions about our experiences with IVIG. The correspondence continued for months, and years later she wrote a piece for the *Huffington Post* about the toll autism took and her effort to find information and pay for treatments for her daughter. She briefly mentioned our email exchanges in the article.

As Amanda says about her connection to other parents through the internet, "I learned how to start emailing strangers like Mary and other mothers, taking extensive notes on everything they tried, including taking down medical specialist's names and taking more notes once we met with those specialists. They [the parents] always had names."

Comparing notes with others online, Amanda realized her daughter was not progressing on the GFCF diet as quickly as most of the other children. Still, she stuck with it, and over a year later the results showed cognitive improvements in her daughter. Amanda explained how it took over ten years for her daughter to reach significant milestones, using intense therapies and interventions. Today, Amanda declares her daughter to be almost recovered.

Amanda epitomizes the seven attributes of a bold parent, never giving up her effort even when it all seemed daunting. When it was decided that IVIG was a course of treatment to consider, Amanda reached out to her celebrity friends to host a benefit in her daughter's honor. The event raised enough money to pay for sixteen IVIG treatments, which Amanda stated had a dramatic impact on Peach. But she could not afford to keep up the treatments. Instead, Amanda continued to educate herself, connect with doctors, network online with other parents, and learn about the next treatments that might improve her daughter's health. All of it worked in varying degrees, even if it took ten years to see what she believes is huge improvement.

In 2014, Peach was accepted into a typical private school where Amanda opted to not disclose anything about autism. Executive functioning challenges and some social impairment remained.

"She can't tell very well when girls are being subtly mean to her; when kids don't want her around. It takes her a while to recognize that a person is really her friend. To the untrained eye, she appears 'normal,'" Amanda said. She ended the year with straight A's and played club soccer in an area known for its competitive sports. No one else knew about her autism, and to Amanda that was perfectly fine.

Chance Encounters Can Lead to Great Things

I have attended many autism conferences over the years, and it seems there is always a "chance" encounter that resonates to the level of "meant to be." One of those chance encounters was Christine Hereen, a professional photographer brought in to take pictures at the first Autism One conference in 2003. She was the mother of a three-year-old boy named Michael who had autism. The conference organizer introduced me to Christine with the thought that I might guide her on starting the GFCF diet, which I was speaking about at the conference.

As Christine recounts, the emails I sent her on how to start the diet were the beginning of her journey. Before she implemented the diet, Christine noted that his behaviors were really "stimming." Within a week of removing dairy, she observed that he no longer rubbed his face on the floor and began to sleep through the night. The gluten removal followed, and more milestones appeared while behaviors began to disappear. She intuitively surrounded herself with like-minded parents who were actively seeking information for their child. In fact, she was one of many parents who counted the connection to the other parents as key to Michael's progress.

"I had to fix whatever was wrong, and if everyone else is doing these things and it's working, I will try them," Christine relayed about immersion into autism treatments. To help her keep track of Michael's progress, Christine started a blog called *Michael's Recovery*, which chronicled each new treatment and how Michael responded, along with the milestones his mother was capturing with her camera. It seemed that wherever Michael went, Christine was there to record the moment with her camera, detailing a legacy of progress.

In 2006, Christine started the first biomedical autism conference in Long Island, New York, and invited a host of speakers to the event. One of the speakers was Julia Berle, who brought her son Baxter to speak about his recovery from autism using chelation, which is used to treat patients who have elevated heavy metal toxicity. This is something most of our children with autism have. Up to that point, all Christine had heard about chelation was how "dangerous" it was. So, hearing a personal account from a mother who had a child recover by using it, Christine decided to look into chelation further. When she hesitated to start treatment because of the annual cost, a relative asked her if it would be worth it if Michael could recover. That comment convinced Christine that she needed to at least give the treatment a try and worry about cost later. As it turned out, her health insurance ended up covering the full price of the chelation, as well as another treatment known as glutathione, which was administered at the same time.

The results were instant. At one time, he had been placed in a separate classroom for children with autism, and as far as Christine was concerned he would probably never move to a different type of class. He was so low functioning that Michael could not respond to ABA therapy. But after starting treatments, Michael quickly began to excel, completely shocking the teaching staff at the local elementary school. He skipped three grades in one day, Christine explained, allowing him to join peers his age in a typical classroom with some academic support.

When the district decided to exempt Michael from taking the state tests in third grade, Christine objected and said he needed to be given the chance to take the test even if he failed it. He didn't fail. In fact, he scored the highest in reading and math in his class, which brought tears of joy to his teacher as she remarked on the progress he had made. Michael had made it through the school year, in spite of predictions he would not progress in the same manner as his peers. "The school did a really good job with him," said Christine of their role in his achievements.

As Michael began to make progress, Christine found there was a need for teaching Michael all over again.

"I think I got to the point with Michael where we healed him, and then it became more a matter of teaching him everything. We just had to show him things in a different way, and keep in mind the way his mind works," said Christine of the relationship with the school district.

When Michael decided to take up the violin, Christine opposed it presuming the instrument would be too difficult for him to learn. But within two months he had mastered playing the violin. He has this infectious and optimistic charisma that his peers respond to. By the time he reached high school, Michael was a popular kid. He eventually went on to become the manager of the baseball team, which had a jersey made just for Michael with his name on the back. He was invited to hang out with the baseball players and was included in their other activities.

For Christine, seeing Michael succeed socially was surreal. When the baseball team handed Michael the game ball after a win, Christine cried with joy because they credited Michael for being their "lucky charm." He was their locker room cheerleader and motivator. He had come a long way from the prospect of having no friends to having many good ones.

She told a story of when Michael was about five, a very spiritual friend taught her how to be positive and visualize making things happen. "He said to me, 'Michael is perfect. You have to start believing in that. It means you are exactly how you are meant to be at this moment. The perfection is he is in the right place.' It was a different version of the word perfect," said Christine. "That was when he started doing better and everything came together. When struggles came up I would keep saying that Michael is perfect, trying to use that word more."

Today Christine would describe high school–aged Michael as ninety percent recovered, and more like a high functioning person with Asperger's. At one time she worried for Michael's future, but now they are planning for college, a career, and one day Michael may decide to get married. All things are possible in every respect of the word.

The Impact We Make

Over the years I have received nice emails of thanks from parents who were grateful that someone was there to get them started, encourage them along the way, or give them advice that proved to be helpful in some way. But none of these emails could compare to a Facebook message I received from a woman named Sarah Carassco of Littleton, Colorado.

> Hi Mary, my name is Sarah and I read your article, "Daniel's Success Story," years ago. I want you to know that it literally saved my son's life. His liver and kidneys were about to shut down when I had him tested for heavy metals. He is doing great, and I'm finally okay myself, lol. From a mother to a mother, thank you. It changed our lives forever. God bless.

The story in *Mothering* magazine on Daniel's story came out in the fall of 2004, and here it was nearly ten years later and I received this message to let me know the impact it had on her son. I had to get the details on what happened to her son, so I called her.

Sarah told a story that would seem unbelievable to many who do not have a child with autism. At three, her son David was so violent with his behaviors that Sarah had been told by two separate people in the same week that he was facing early residential placement. They warned her that he would become too much for her to handle, and that he presented a threat to her one-year-old infant. She describes how his behaviors were so bad that the doctors refused to give him an autism diagnosis and were leaning in the direction of psychosis without explanation. She scheduled an appointment with a pharmacology clinic in preparation for a possible move to residential placement.

"He was undiagnosable because he was so severe. There are kids who are severe, but they all pale in comparison. He was extremely violent all day. I didn't sleep for three to four hours a night until he was five," Sarah recounts of that time.

As a newly separated mother trying to juggle her family, her job, and find answers for her son, she found herself at a very low point in her life. Facing the prospect of losing her son, she prayed for answers and guidance on how to help him. As she describes the sequence of events, it was the next day that her son's occupational therapist handed her a photocopy of the *Mothering* magazine article that had just come out that month. This changed Sarah's entire perspective on the possibilities.

Sarah said that after she read the story, she followed the sidebar section of what I suggested were the first steps to take. Top of the list was to start the GFCF diet. Although I recommended implementing the diet in stages, Sarah was desperate and anguished. She felt that time was not on their side. After a four-hour trip to the grocery store where she read every label, she decided to start the diet "cold turkey," meaning fully and all at once. Within three weeks the violent behavior had decreased by half. He had better eye contact and his extreme rages were virtually gone. She had further tests done which confirmed he had significant food allergies and she removed those foods too.

Even the preschool noticed the significant difference in David, as did Sarah's parents. When she took him for the appointment with the pharmacology clinic, the doctors were perplexed as to why she was even there with David. Clearly, the child in front of them was not in need of their services since he had no discernible violent behaviors, which Sarah took as validation for the path they were on.

"Everything I was witnessing was a miracle. Three months into the diet I woke up and he was staring at me. Then he signed I love you," Sarah said.

In the meantime, her mother researched and found a local DAN doctor, and scheduled an appointment for a couple months later in January 2005. Shortly after the initial visit where blood labs were drawn, Sarah received an anxious phone call from the doctor. Realizing a call from a doctor was probably not good news, she asked if she could call him after work when she would be more prepared to deal with the information. When she did call him back his voice was grave. He explained that her son's heavy metal levels were the worst he had ever seen, and his kidneys and liver panel showed they were close to shutting down. He needed to send a nurse over to the house to begin chelation treatments, starting that night.

As Sarah came to grips with the idea that her son could have died, she began an intensely emotional and physical journey to heal him. Chelation continued for five months, as did other treatments to help heal his compromised immune system.

"The most notable change in our life is that, as his mother, I knew he didn't feel well," reflected Sarah. "Once we got through the chelation, all of those symptoms were gone. He was looking at me, could communicate, and was sitting better in school. When you look at his school records, there was a definite change there. He went from the worst behaved kid in class to the best behaved kid in class."

Sarah describes David, now in his teens, as having mid- to high-functioning autism. While he is two years behind on most subjects, he reads at grade level. But his life is still a miracle to her.

"I honestly think he will be fine. We just continue to do more interventions and therapy constantly," said Sarah of David's future. "I think when it comes to autism, if we can teach him adequate social skills then he will be fine. He is definitely in there and he understands everything that is going on around him."

Looking back on the serendipitous moment when the magazine story came to her at the time it did, Sarah pauses before adding, "It changed the course of our lives." She now looks ahead at what still needs to be done for the families who still need information to change the course of their lives, and the health of their children. "We can't get to millions right now. So I think we have to keep the emphasis on individuals."

Indeed we do.

When the Parents Are Doctors

The thing about attending so many conferences is that, after a while, you find that many of your best information sessions happen in the hallway conversations between presentations. So, as I was heading to yet another presentation by a well-known physician, I lingered a bit to check out the vendor booths that lined the exhibit area. At one of these booths was a cheery, pretty woman from Branson, Missouri, named Dr. Leah Parker who spoke with a strong southern accent. We immediately liked each other. What was meant to be a quick information-only question turned into a conversation that lasted the duration of the speaker's presentation. And it seemed that I kept running into Leah wherever I went, until we finally decided to just sit and have a lengthy chat about what led her to become a doctor of naturopathic medicine after being a traditional medicine nurse.

As Leah described her journey, it all began to sound familiar: a desperate mother needing answers for her child and disillusioned with traditional medical approaches, she decided to seek answers in other areas. It was the path—the script if you will—we all seemed to be following.

She went on to detail how her now twenty-year-old daughter had reacted badly to all of the vaccines she had received as an infant, including coming down with measles from the MMR. "Her immune system was severely compromised," related Leah. Her daughter had chronic illnesses, dark circles under her eyes, stridor respiratory reactions, and inflamed kidneys. Subsequent tests revealed that her daughter was severely allergic to everything she was eating, which was a clear signal to Leah that her daughter had "leaky gut" syndrome.

Diagnosed at five with severe ADHD, the doctors put her on medication that left the girl exhausted and zombie-like. So the parents stopped the medication, home schooled their daughter, and started researching for alternative answers.

"I started to look for a doctor but there was not anyone. In Branson, little was known about autism. If it is not in their lives, they don't know about it," Leah said. Later when her son was diagnosed with autism, the need for this kind of doctor became more acute. As a registered nurse, the idea began to cross her mind that she may need to go back to school to study the immune system's connection to autism.

She prayed for answers as her daughter's symptoms worsened, begging God to guide her. "I was standing in line to get yet another prescription and I kept being guided to 'herbs.'

Of course, they don't teach you anything about that in nursing school," Leah said, with emphasis on the "of course" part.

Several days later, her basement flooded and a local plumber was called to fix it. The project took a full three days for the repair. During that time, the plumber and Leah struck up a conversation on health issues, with the plumber telling Leah that without a doubt her daughter's immune system had been compromised by the vaccines. Being disdainful of vaccine skeptics, she asked for credible information to back his assertions that vaccines could be harmful. The next day he brought back information from a Christian organization known as Concerned Women for America, which was the first bit of evidence that caused Leah to begin doing her own investigation on the side effects of vaccines.

The research she compiled over the next six months turned into a hundred and fifty page paper, which she eventually used when she decided to enter naturopathic medical school. It took her some time as a medical professional to accept that her daughter's chronic illness was related to vaccine injury, but once she did, it set her off in a different direction of understanding that would change the course of her life.

"This is not just about autism," she clarified. "This is about chronic childhood disease, including ADD, ADHD, Type 1 diabetes, juvenile rheumatoid arthritis, childhood cancer, allergies, and asthma." And to Leah, it isn't just vaccines causing harm to our children; she also took aim at pesticides, food additives, and other environmental triggers. It was her contention that the vaccine schedule needed to be delayed for two years, and that more had to be done to address the mother's body burden before pregnancy, including removing amalgam fillings.

As she set about healing the immune systems of her children, she realized that other families were also in need of the same information. So, when she became a naturopathic medical doctor, she dedicated her practice to reaching those who would not usually begin the healing journey because they could not afford it. "My goal was to find a way to treat these kids without breaking the bank. So many people cannot afford it, so they do nothing."

She charges a nominal amount for a consultation. It's a ministry, a calling, a passion to reach the parent of the ill child and provide them with information, hope, and treatments that are helpful, all without being hugely expensive. And several of her patients have gone on to recover from autism.

"I am really trying to work with people and get them help here. The majority cannot afford biomedical treatment and the kid is not going to get help," she adds.

Her own children are improving through dietary and immune system interventions, but Leah is cautious on how she describes them. She is reluctant to use the word "recovered," instead opting for "repair mode" as a more accurate description for how they are doing.

She finally adds with a laugh, "Thank God I got educated!"

Creating Our Own Miracles

I met Tracey when she and her family relocated to our town from Germany. As a military family they were used to changes and ensured that their children got involved with the local scouts and church, which is where I was first introduced to Tracey. Tracey's daughter and Theresa became friends and eventually so did Tracey and I. One day, we struck up a conversation after she told me about her then eight-year-old son Michael who had been diagnosed with autism in Germany five years earlier. I briefly shared with her our story of Daniel's recovery and we agreed to meet later to discuss it further.

Over coffee at a local café, we began to talk in-depth about autism treatment options, which astounded Tracey who had not heard that autism could be treated. Instead, she thought her only remedy for autism was to rely on a "miracle" for Michael so that he would improve, or recover. I looked at Tracey and said, "You need to go create the miracle. Let me show you how." We began to talk regularly on how to implement diet changes and choose physicians to go to for further answers.

Something about Michael, and Tracey's effort to help him, felt personal. I think it was because she was my friend and lived in my town, or because I saw in Michael many of the traits that used to exist in Daniel. Either way, I knew she would not have to navigate this path alone. With the right tools, I knew Tracey would make it happen. As I laid out the reasons to consider dietary changes, she mentioned that Michael just seemed spacey, which I told her was a direct result from the foods he was eating. It was a type of opioid effect, I explained, which created a brain fog of sorts. She would later tell me, "I went with GFCF and soy-free diet, and within a few months I noticed Michael was not as spacey. He seemed to check back in."

Since Tracey's husband was not going to be available, I agreed to attend the follow-up appointment with the physician to go over the result of the labs. I braced Tracey for what the labs may indicate and a potential course of treatment, depending on the outcome. As it turned out, the labs indicated that Michael had significant levels of lead, which Tracey believed was from military housing contamination, and would benefit from chelation therapy. He also presented with multiple food allergies and intolerances to virtually everything he was eating. The one thing he didn't present with was an overgrowth of yeast, which was a good thing since chelation would not begin until yeast was under control. During the doctor's appointment I brought up the possibility of Michael benefiting from glutathione and vitamin C, and asked if Tracey should consider adding these to the chelation cocktail since they tended to work synergistically. Tracey and the physician thought it was a good idea and ordered the combination.

In the meantime, Tracey had become a proficient researcher. While her son received the chelation therapy, she continued to look into other treatment modalities and physicians as they began to prepare for their next military-family move. The thread of possibilities had been pulled by Tracey and she was going to continue to unravel the answers for Michael.

The next therapy she looked into was a sound therapy to improve his auditory processing delay, which is common in children with autism.

"My goal for him was simple. I wanted him to be invited to a birthday party. It had been years since he had been invited to one, and I know a portion of that was moving with the military. The bigger picture was that I wanted him to be interacting with friends," Tracey remarked. The sound therapy began to make a profound difference in Michael's ability to process what he was hearing, allowing him to connect more easily to his peers. When Tracey and I met before she moved, we talked about how she needed to raise the bar on expectations for Michael's achievements in the classroom since he was making increasing and amazing strides. When he was assigned to a new school after the move to Michigan, Michael began to not need some of his supports in the classroom because he was beginning to make progress at grade level.

"They actually called me a week after school and asked where the boy on the IEP was because Mike was not what they were expecting. That is when I knew I was on the right track to recovery. Mike wasn't the boy on the IEP anymore," Tracey added.

Not long after, the family made yet one more move to Texas, and Tracey determined it was time to get a handle on his significant food allergies. For this next therapy she consulted with a local homeopathic doctor whom she worked with for over a year, which Tracey credits with clearing the final immune system hurdle, allowing Michael to overcome his food allergies.

Today, Michael is a teen on his way to achieving Eagle Scout rank in his local troop. He is performing academically at grade level and is considered virtually indiscernible from his typical peers. That's the miracle that she prayed for.

When Success Is Defined by the Milestones

Carolyn Gammicchia wasn't sure what recovery would look like for her son Nick, nor was she banking on it. But she did want him to be able to function somewhat independently and contribute to society. It's a goal for most parents of special needs children to know that their child can participate in the world, ideally independently.

The Gammicchias are a close-knit family. Andrew is a police officer, while Carolyn is a retired police officer who happens to run an autism non-profit called L.E.A.N. On Us, that stands for Law Enforcement Awareness Network, which provides information to law enforcement agencies to understand and serve individuals in their communities affected by mental illness and hidden disabilities. Who better to inform police officers on autism and other disabilities than another police officer who has a child with autism?

Their two adult sons are Alex and Nick, both in college. Nick has autism that at one time was so severe that the idea that he would one day attend college was a distant dream belonging to someone else, as far as Carolyn was concerned. But she was also committed to finding solutions for Nick to be able to succeed at any level; including starting programs in her local school district because nothing existed until Nick arrived needing the services.

When Nick's behaviors escalated when he was in grade school, Carolyn made the decision to retire from police work and focus on his needs. She was determined to keep Nick safe and out of group homes, without medication. She started Nick with Relationship Development Intervention (RDI) which is a behavior therapy to build up his social skills. She also simplified the home routine, added in massage therapy, changed his diet, and over a period of six weeks the effort to get his behaviors under control was successful. It was all done without medication.

Carolyn is a goal-oriented person, but she wants to ensure that her life is otherwise simplified. It's within that context that the Gammicchias made a conscious decision to forego attachments to material things and focus on connecting to the world around them by traveling—a lot! On their many trips to Europe, the family learned to navigate public transportation in a variety of countries, which helped build confidence in Nick. There are no predictable routines when you travel abroad, which is why Nick was challenged to be flexible.

"Nick used to study the languages of the countries we would visit. You are acclimating to the culture while you are in an environment where you don't know the expectation," said Carolyn with a glimmer of pride.

When the family traveled to Hawaii, Nick was in a life-threatening situation that could have led to panic. Only, he didn't panic and did exactly what he needed to do to keep calm and get out of the crisis. That was when Carolyn knew Nick was going to be just fine. He would find his way in the world and felt confident that he could adapt in a tough moment.

"It framed in us what we were looking for in Nick's future. It actually validated what we had worked so hard for him to be able to do," reflected Carolyn.

When Nick was in high school, he decided that he wanted to go to college, especially after watching Alex graduate and head off. Nick always wanted to do the things Alex did, and now that included college. This meant that the plan for this achievement was going to have to rely on Carolyn's effort to create the program at the high school for Nick, as she had all the years before. Carolyn had to find the way for Nick to receive his diploma, not just a certificate. A "bridge" model was created at the school that allowed Nick to simultaneously take college and high school courses to help him transition to college-level work.

At one point, all of the Gammicchias were enrolled at the same time in the same college, taking individual courses on the way to their degrees. When Nick took his first college math class, Carolyn sat in the back of the class watching how he would do. But her concern was reduced when the professor and his scribing aid told her that Nick was fine and didn't need any additional intervention. He was right on par with his college peers. Carolyn breathed a sigh of relief, and utter disbelief.

"I never thought he would go to college," said Carolyn. "When he was in elementary school, I thought he would never make it in junior high. Then he went to high school. And now college!" As a matter of philosophy about Nick's potential, Carolyn adds, "We got rid of the box because we didn't want any limitations at all." Carolyn also insisted that part of Nick's growth involved allowing him to fail. When he struggled in an English class and failed it, she didn't interfere, but he eventually improved and passed the class the next time he took it.

The RDI therapy paid off too, because, as Carolyn describes, Nick is now the life of the party. When high school prom came along, Nick insisted on going stag in order to be able to dance with more girls. When the night was over, the dance tally was thirty-six girls, six of whom kissed him. "I would have never thought that he would be the life of the party, and he was," said Carolyn with a laugh.

When he graduates with his degree in art, Nick plans to work in the film industry writing screenplays and illustrating storyboards. No doubt he is someone we will be hearing more about one day. He doesn't know there are supposed to be limitations for him, which is the very reason why he will succeed.

Because What We Do as Caregivers Matters

Jennifer Barsamian and I seem to have run parallel lives over the past decade. Both of us have a son the same age who is considered recovered. We have also continued to mentor in the community, and we have both at one point stepped away from the battle in order to regroup. For Jennifer, dropping out of the community also came about because her son needed her attention all over again. That's the thing about recovered children and their parents. We are never, ever done. For Jennifer, her son was considered recovered so they stopped most of his interventions, only to have him regress into obsessive-compulsive behaviors.

"It was right back down again," Jennifer said of that time in their lives when her son, then five years old, began to regress all over again. Jennifer thought, "I can't put this kid out there as recovered. It has been an up-and-down battle for us for years. I am always waiting for the other shoe to fall."

I completely understood this feeling. It carries with it a level of PTSD to feel your child slipping back into former behaviors and health patterns, or maybe new health issues come up. It grips you at the core and you revert back to the parent you thought you would never have to be again. As Jennifer describes her feelings, "I am constantly vigilant. My fear is that he is so chemically sensitive that he is going to fall apart again." Even planning for college involves investigating whether there are chemical-free dorm rooms.

But the fact that he is cognitively and in all other ways ready to go to college is a milestone. Besides diet, Jennifer says that that the treatments that helped her son the most were GcMAF, sauna, and hyperbaric oxygen (HBOT). GcMAF is a protein the body makes that acts as a "director" of the immune system. All three therapies combined helped to detox the body and repair his damaged immune system.

Jennifer describes how for the first two weeks of his life he was lovely. He slept, ate, and was calm. Then, at two weeks, he received his first vaccine, the hepatitis B vaccine, and after that he was a shrieking mess of colic, projectile vomit, gas, and diarrhea. If he wasn't sleeping or nursing he was screaming, and this went on for months.

He was diagnosed at three with autism, which Jennifer said took her by surprise. He was one of those "genius" babies that could recite the alphabet at nine months, he was verbal and had a memory. But he was not socially engaged and didn't point to anything until he was seven years old. He lined up his toys, scripted from the television, but had no original thought. But for Jennifer and her husband, the behaviors were not as much of an issue as the rest of his chronic health problems, including fevers, twenty ear infections in the first year of his life, pneumonia, and respiratory issues. He was put on repeated rounds of antibiotics, yet he continued to get sicker.

Motivated by her son's spiraling health, she implemented a variety of dietary interventions and other treatments. But Jennifer fell into the same trap many of us do. Feeling like she was battling the enigma of "time," she and her husband started their son on so many treatment modalities at once that they were not sure what was working. Something was, however, because he began to slowly get better.

When thinking of the various therapies she and her husband considered trying, Jennifer can recall how often she would think, "'Oh my gosh, this is it.' Only it was never it; just the next step in the progression." But each step added up so that by his teens he was indistinguishable from his peers. He went on to become a top soccer player in spite of his former gross motor deficits. He is still on dietary intervention and mindful of what he needs to continue to do the rest of his life to maintain his health. It seems almost unfair to have a boy so aware of his tenuous health, but it is a small price to pay for the chance to live the life that at one time was thought impossible.

For Jennifer, the dream of a full life for her son with autism became a reality. As Jennifer relates, "I have never seen a kid do biomedical interventions and not see some improvement on some level. My son improved because of what we did. Doctors need to give us parents the benefit of the doubt on what is working. Improvement is possible."

Yes, and so is recovery.

Recovered and Now a Customer Liaison

Just as I was ready to forward the manuscript of this book to the publisher, I learned of a young man in his twenties who was recovered and working as an engineer for a large aerospace company as a *customer liaison* (read: interfacing with customers on behalf of the company). I contacted the publisher to ask for a little more time on the manuscript because I wanted to include the story of this family whose hurdles must have been tremendous, and yet they prevailed. Today's parents have no idea how much information is available compared to a decade ago, let alone two decades ago. That is why this story was important to include.

Marcia Hinds and I have decided we were either sisters in a past life or generals on the battlefield together. As mothers of sons who have overcome autism, and having both helped other parents find answers for their children, we were tripping over each other with excitement in our first conversation.

"How is it I have not met you before?" was my first question to Marcia, to which Marcia piped up that we had to be sisters somewhere before. She then added that, because her son was older than mine, we were not on the journey at the same time and so did not run into each other online or in person.

Marcia wrote a book about her son's recovery called *I Know You're In There*. It was a page-turner account of her son's spiraling behaviors and diagnosis, followed by finding the answers through diet and treatments. What I marveled at most was how she did not mince words, calling out doctors, therapists, and school staff by name for both the good and the bad side of how they handled Ryan. A lot of autism books are a tough read for me because I am always looking for the lines of hope in the text. Marcia's book was littered with both hope and chutzpah. If you had to have a poster child for exuding the seven attributes, Marcia's face would be there.

It was evident why Ryan recovered. His mother and father never gave up. Ever. In fact, she tells me he was still affected in his teens but she kept up with treatments, diet, and therapies until he no longer needed them as a young adult. But this was a long way from the prognosis that one doctor declared that they should just hope he can be functional enough to work in a basement away from people as an adult. What Marcia and her husband Frank also did was write a lot of letters to doctors, therapists, and everyone in between to let them know how their interaction with her, her husband, or her son affected them, whether it was positive or not. Perhaps it was their way of venting their outrage at the ignorance exhibited by the experts who took away hope with their dismal prognosis over Ryan's future.

Instead of having a bleak future, Ryan went on to be accepted into a number of top colleges and universities, choosing a major university in the same state to pursue a degree in engineering, where he graduated with honors.

What I especially liked about Marcia and her book is that she echoes what this book also says: our children can experience improved health and even recovery with the right medical treatments, dietary changes, educational supports, and therapies. Most will, at the very least, improve, but that does not mean every child will. But it is still worth the parents' effort to at least try to find the possibilities.

Marcia adds in her book:

> I want more children to recover. There are too many kids not getting what they need. Valuable time is lost when parents have to wade through massive amounts of information and misinformation to help their child. And, it is difficult to know when it is the right decision to go against the ideas of our trusted, well-meaning doctors. It has taken way too much time to change minds and shift the paradigm from autism as a psychiatric disorder to autism as a treatable medical condition.

Marcia goes on to say that, while her son is recovered, he is not cured, because of the medications he must rely on to help his immune system work. Likewise, I say the same about Daniel:

recovery is not the same thing as cured. Still, we are grateful, and I am glad to know Marcia and I are on the battlefield together once again.

Raun Kaufman

When Daniel lost his diagnosis in 2003, I was unsure what exactly that meant. Besides the perpetual vigilance on his health that overtook my own psyche, I wondered what life in adulthood would look like for him. So I emailed Raun Kaufman, who is by all accounts a "rock star" to autism parents because he is considered one of the first to recover from autism. More importantly, he was still involved in the community as the CEO and current Director of Global Education for the non-profit Autism Treatment Center of America™ located in Sheffield, Massachusetts.

I knew about Raun's story just from hanging out with parents who were looking for answers. His name and story was mentioned with such regularity that you had the impression his fame would mean that he would have more than his share of fan mail and would probably not reply to an email from one more mother asking for information. But he did. I asked him what his life was like today and what I should look forward to for my son's future. Raun could not have been more gracious with his reply, detailing his "normal" life and encouraging me to not set limits on our son's future (in a nutshell).

Fast forward a decade and Raun and I are now both living in Massachusetts and we both have books coming out on the idea that children with autism are treatable and can improve or recover. I found out that Raun's book, *Autism Breakthrough*, was coming out in April 2014 and so I contacted the Autism Treatment Center™ to see if we could have Raun come speak to the TACA Massachusetts families. It's one thing to hear from another parent about recovery; it is entirely something else to hear from the recovered and successful adult.

Raun was born in 1973 to Barry and Samahria Kaufman. By the age of two, Raun was diagnosed with severe autism and the Kaufman's were told that it was incurable and lifelong. The words "institution" and "group home" were thrown in for good measure. Instead of accepting the prognosis for their child, they

created a home-based program for Raun. They began by enthu-
siastically "joining" him in his stimming behaviors of spinning
plates and other rituals. Then once they had his willing engage-
ment they helped him interact more and more by using games
and activities they developed based upon Raun's own motiva-
tions and interests. Raun's parents intuitively gravitated to what
they believed he needed, and so they started him with other
therapies when they believed he was ready to engage in the
process.

Raun began to thrive, exceeding all the doctors' expectations. Raun's parents had, or developed, the seven attributes of
the bold parent. They tapped especially into optimism and held
on to it with a grit of determination that is mind-blowing when
you realize how alone they must have felt. They were truly
the pioneers of the *possible* in autism. Knowing that this home-
based, child-centered philosophy and therapy (given the name
Son-Rise®) was something other parents would benefit from,
Raun's dad Barry wrote a book, published in 1976, called *Son-
Rise* (now called *Son Rise: A Miracle Continues*), a book about the
triumph over autism. Later, a TV movie was made in 1979 called
Son-Rise: A Miracle of Love.

Rather than settle for the gloomy prognosis, the Kaufmans
reached for the brass ring and achieved it. Raun was successful
and highly social in high school, and then went on to graduate
from Brown University with a degree in Biomedical Ethics. Now
you know why his story was so compelling to so many of us who
dared for the same outcome for our children.

When Raun spoke at the TACA meeting, I watched his
animated and poised delivery with a measure of "Gee, I hope
Daniel is this charismatic one day." He was funny, personable,
confident, and in all ways a delight to this group. Later, a few of
the parent volunteers and I took Raun to lunch as a thank you,
and to get to know him better. We sat for the next two hours
laughing and listening, sharing a similar philosophy that the
sky is the limit for the future of our children, which is why we
quickly became friends.

As I was winding down this last chapter of the book, I suddenly realized he needed to be in it. Calling him, I knew the first

question was the last one I had emailed him over a decade ago: what does recovery mean?

"I consider someone fully recovered when they are not only free of outward symptoms but they are recovered on the inside too," said Raun. "They don't have to work extra hard in social situations and they are not secretly holding themselves back from repetitive behaviors."

But he wanted to be sure to suggest that victory over autism does not only look like full recovery. He added, "Children recover or improve at varying levels. The main thing is not to put the limits on our children ahead of time. What I feel strongly about is that there are no time limits on what a child or adult can do." Adults? "Yes, even adults," he said while going on to explain that a twenty-six-year-old today may achieve skills later in life. "We still have no idea what that person is going to be like at thirty-two [and beyond]," Raun said with emphasis on the words "no idea."

Raun elaborated that there is a huge shift happening in the understanding of autism and the idea that it can be treated, although there is still need for a greater awareness to seep into our psyche as a community. He explained that what he sees is this reluctance in professional society to offer parents the simplest of hope, as though it is more "humane" for parents to not be given "false hope." What he has tried to do in his numerous lectures and in his book is to suggest that the future for the child is not known, so don't predetermine what it is supposed to be.

When asked what he says to parents in his lectures when they are faced with the prospect of a dismal future for their child, Raun decided to give me bullet points as part of the answer.

1. Don't believe anyone that predicts some gloomy outcome for your kid.

2. The most powerful and loving place to start is by "embracing where your child is right now." This gives you your best shot at connecting with your child.

3. Know that, as a parent, you have what it takes to help your child. Parents are told "Oh, you're just a mom." There are all these messages that we are told as parents

we are not capable. You have what it takes to make a gigantic difference in your child's life.

So many of us are saying the same things about hope, recovery, and a bright future ahead for our children that it seems indicative that Raun is right. No one knows the future, so don't limit the possibilities for our kids. I will add that no one knows the future, but we sure as heck can try to create it.

Implementing the GFCF Diet in 10 Easy Weeks

What is gluten? Proteins found in the plant kingdom: wheat, oats, barley, rye, triticale, spelt, kamut, and all derivatives such as malt, grain starches, hydrolyzed vegetable plant proteins, textured vegetable proteins, grain vinegars, soy sauce, grain alcohols, flavorings, and the binders and fillers found in vitamins and medications.

What is casein? A phosphoprotein of milk, which has a molecular structure similar to gluten and includes:
- Milk
- Butter
- Cheese
- Yogurt
- Ice cream
- Creams
- Caseinate
- Pediasure

What is leaky gut? Many of our kids (and adults) have gastro-intestinal disorders believed to be caused by an insult to the immune system, which contributes to the gluten and casein proteins breakdown of the intestinal wall. Proteins go through a permeable gut wall and cross the blood/brain barrier, causing many of the autism symptoms. These include:

- Clouded mental function
- Insomnia
- Diarrhea
- Impaired social connection
- Blocking of pain messages
- Dilated pupils
- Crave opioid effect from food

But my child only eats five foods: Yes, I know. And they are usually chicken nuggets, milk, cheese, french fries, and a chip of some sort. All gluten and casein foods. This is why I tell parents that their child is addicted to the effect of the foods, not the flavors, and must be treated as though it is a "narcotic" for them. We would no more hand a candy bar to a child diagnosed with diabetes or a slice of bread to a child with celiac; so too we must be cognizant of how these proteins impact our children with leaky gut and autism.

Before beginning dietary intervention: Understand you are beginning a lifestyle change that will take a lifetime if done correctly. What many doctors who treat autism do not understand is that gluten and casein are not IgG intolerance foods that can eventually be returned to the diet. They are the proteins that break down the mucosa lining of the gut wall, so even after a child is recovered from autism they must remain on the diet or risk regression. They may not necessarily revert back into autism, but they may develop some other autoimmune or mental health disorder. I have met a number of families whose recovered child gave up the diet and other interventions, only to have a new symptom or disorder appear. It is the worst feeling to see your child, who you considered to be recovered, revert back to former behaviors or have a new health concern. Remember, our children are the pioneers in the whole idea that children can recover from autism. So, anything I mention here on what to look out for does not necessarily have a study attached to it, just quite a few anecdotes from the parents who have gone before, including me.

Don't try to tackle the full ten weeks all at once (if possible). I have seen some children go through significant withdrawals where they would seek out the gluten/casein proteins in non-edible items like Play-Doh, licking envelopes, or eating toothpaste just to get the opioid effect back in their body. My own son would throw tantrums and hang off the refrigerator door begging for milk. But by sticking with it, past my own angst over having to do the diet, our son recovered in large part because of it. He remains healthy today.

Also, by breaking out the diet into ten weeks you create a sense of confidence that cascades into the next decisions you will be making, especially when you begin to see the changes in your child. If you want to move the calendar up quicker, do so after the second week.

Cross contamination considerations: In the early part of the diet, it is wise to follow the no cross contamination rule, especially after the ten week diet has been fully implemented. In other words, if the label on the item tells you the product may be cross contaminated with a potential allergen (intolerance), then avoid the product entirely. If you cook gluten foods or with ingredients, be sure to avoid cross contamination with foods your child would eat. If your child goes after the harmful foods or ingredients in a quest to get them back in the body, then they need to be removed from the house for a period of time or for good.

When Daniel got a hold of just a swath of butter and a nibble of a gluten cookie, we saw the reaction in him for a week. It typically takes about two days to show up in the child in the mode of a delayed reaction of cognition and/or behaviors. So avoid any and all prospect of the offending foods getting in to your child. Also, if your child is one of those who waits to eat until they can eat the gluten/casein foods, then you will need to speed up the diet after the second week to be fully gluten/casein free.

What's the deal with soy? Soy is similar in molecular structure to casein, so it is best to avoid it, especially in larger amounts like milk and ice cream. For us, we had to remove soy altogether for years while his gut healed since it was the main culprit to some of his gut issues. As he got older and his gut was healed, we were able to add soy back in as a sub-ingredient only, not as a main item. He no longer had an intolerance indicated on his IgG panel either. However, gluten and casein are still removed from his diet, and will continue to be.

Week 1 and 2:
- Remove all milk-based products
- Do not replace with soy milk or yogurt. Instead, replace with rice milk, coconut milk, almond milk or Dari-free, non-dairy margarines, and cheese (no whey as an ingredient).
- Add in a calcium/magnesium supplement to avoid eye stimming and more sleep problems.
- During these two weeks, read the book *Special Diets for Special Kids* by Lisa Lewis to understand the science behind the diet, and find some creative kid-friendly recipes to get started.
- Stock up on gluten-free foods.
- Buy ready to eat and package mixes only in the beginning. Go easy on yourself during this transition period and avoid complicated recipes with multiple ingredients you do not ordinarily have on hand. That will come later once you have gotten further into the diet transition.

Week 3
Find five GFCF foods that your child will eat for breakfast, and serve it.
- Frozen GFCF waffles and real maple syrup
- Bacon and eggs (GFCF bacon, preferably uncured) and hash browns like Cascadian Farms
- Cream of Rice cereal
- Gluten-free oatmeal
- Nature's Path organic gluten/casein-free cereals (they have quite a few)
- Envirokids cereals
- GFCF pancakes (Trader Joe's sells a frozen version, or you can make your own from a quick mix)
- Earth Balance margarine is a good butter replacement (purchase the soy free version, if possible)

Week 4

Find five GFCF foods your child will eat for lunch and serve it, maintaining the GFCF breakfast choices.

- GFCF and soy-free hot dog (preferably an uncured brand) with or without a GFCF bun.
- Chicken or turkey hot dogs with or without a GFCF bun.
- Corn chips or a gluten-free tortilla chip (most chips are dairy free unless they have a milk-based flavor ingredient).
- Potato chip (again, just check for the allergen information on the label to see if the brand is okay to use).
- Organic french fries that can be baked. Cascadian Farm or another brand that is similar will suffice. Avoid any brand with caramel coloring since it may be a gluten.
- Lunch meats such as Applegate brand, preferably without sulfites.
- Avoid providing too much juice in place of milk since the extra sugar may exacerbate an underlying yeast overgrowth (which many of our kids have as part of the leaky gut). Best to stick with plain water, or water down the juice significantly in the early stages of the diet.

Week 5

Find five foods your child will eat for dinner, and serve it, maintaining the breakfast and lunch choices. Truthfully, dinner is the easiest meal to serve GFCF for the whole family since it typically consists of a protein, starch, and a vegetable. Just prepare without gluten/casein or soy ingredients and the meal is perfect for everyone.

- Rice-, corn-, or quinoa-based pasta, along with a gluten-free spaghetti sauce. Usually, most organic brands of jarred pasta sauce are gluten free. Just check the label for ingredients and cross contamination.
- Roasted chicken, baked potatoes, vegetables
- Hamburgers with organic baked french fries, vegetables
- Homemade chicken nuggets prepared GFCF
- Any breakfast or lunch item for dinner

Week 6
Replace all snack items with GFCF and soy-free versions.
- GFCF pretzels and other chips
- Popcorn (look for organic non-microwave versions, if possible)
- Fresh fruit
- Enjoy Life Foods cookies and snacks
- Envirokids snack bars
- Glutino snack foods

Week 7
Replace all soaps, shampoos, toothpaste, laundry detergent, lotions, sunscreens, medications, and vitamins to be fully GFCF. Many of your regular brands may already be GFCF. To check if your brand is okay to use, go to www.GFCFDiet.com. If you would like to take it further and replace these products for fully safe and environmentally friendly brands, go to Environmental Working Group at www.ewg.org.

Week 8
Replace all classroom supplies that contain gluten such as Play-Doh and stickers. Many schools have become significantly aware of the dangers of potential allergens and are quick to assist this kind of change. A helpful guide for teachers can be found on www.tacanow.org, under family resources. I offered to replace many of these supplies and in all other ways helped the teacher to avoid having these contaminants in the classroom. It would also help to have GFCF treats on hand in the event of an unplanned party where the rest of the children are served regular treats.

Week 9
Begin making GFCF snacks and meals from ingredients you have on hand at all times. Again, dinner is the easiest transition to this kind of change in how you perceive your new cooking lifestyle. Try your hand at stir fries, freshly baked foods, and even organic ingredients. The more you move to this healthier form for your child with autism, the more the rest of the family will benefit.

Week 10

Begin making GFCF snacks and meals using flours and ingredients you would not ordinarily have on hand, including flours like tapioca flour and starch, potato flour and starch, rice flour, all purpose GFCF flour, sorghum flour, xanthum gum, coconut flour, coconut oil, and sea salt. For sugar, many of us move in the direction of eliminating sugars as much as possible or seek out alternative forms of sweeteners like stevia and coconut sugar (you need to do your research on this before deciding on switching sweeteners). Avoid ALL artificial sweeteners.

What else?

Dietary intervention, especially GFCF, is just the beginning of changes you will make in the quest to get your child well. But it is the crucially important *first* step.

- Become educated on why to do the diet so that you can understand why it is necessary to make these changes.
- A little bit WILL hurt. Avoid the idea that a little here or there is okay to do as long as you are mostly GFCF. Even a smidge means your child is potentially reacting to the gluten and the casein, in particular, so these need to be avoided at all times.
- Educate your spouse on the GFCF diet if necessary, and include your partner in on the decisions and why these changes are necessary for the child and beneficial for the family.
- Educate other family members and those in close contact with your child and insist that your child not be fed the harmful foods.
- Eating out is completely doable for GFCF. Because gluten has become problematic for many Americans, restaurants have become wise and are providing gluten-free menus. You just need to further avoid the dairy ingredients and other allergens on the menu as well.
- Traveling with a child with a GFCF diet in place is easy with the proper planning, including checking with the hotel on arrangements to have GFCF foods on hand

before your arrival. Theme parks will also list their allergen friendly foods and places to get them on their websites.

- Avoid fast food restaurants if possible. The quality and the ingredients in these foods are questionable for all of us, especially for a child with a compromised immune system and gut issues.
- Purchase organic foods whenever you can. The more you can eliminate toxins from your child the better.
- DO NOT consider digestive enzymes as a replacement for implementing the diet. There are many reasons for this, mostly because digestive enzymes are not a long-term answer but a short-term bandage. Use digestive enzymes as a supplement to help heal the gut, on top of implementing diet and other treatments.

Steps to take to begin healing the gut, the brain, and the immune system.
- GFCF and soy-free diet
- IgG food sensitivity removal
- Antifungals and probiotics
- Biomedical treatments
- Digestive enzymes
- Find a MAPS or functional medicine doctor to begin testing for appropriate treatments

Resources

General Information Resources
- Talk About Curing Autism – www.tacanow.org
- Autism One conference – www.autismone.org
- Autism Research Institute – www.autism.com
- National Autism Association – www.nationalautismasso-ciation.org
- Generation Rescue – www.generationrescue.org
- Thinking Moms Revolutions – www.thinkingmoms-revolution.com
- Autism is Medical – www.autismismedical.com
- Safeminds – www.safeminds.org
- Unlocking Autism – www.unlockingautism.org
- Lenny Schafer Report – www.sarnet.org
- The Pfeiffer Institute – www.hriptc.org
- Dana's View – www.danasview.net
- Autism Society of America – www.autism-society.org
- US Autism/Asperger Association – www.usautism.org
- Fearless Parent – www.fearlessparent.org
- Autism Speaks – www.autismspeaks.org

General Information for Biomedical Treatments and Therapies
- General Overview – www.tacanow.org/tag/medical/
- General Overview – www.autism.com
- General Overview – www.generationrescue.org
- General Overview – www.autismone.org
- Physician/Parent perspective – www.biomedicaltreat-mentforautism.com

Behavior Therapies
- Lovaas Therapy – www.behavior-analysis.org

- Floortime – www.stanleygreenspan.com
- Rapid Response – www.halo-soma.org
- Verbal Behavior – www.carboneclinic.com
- Verbal Behavior Institute – www.teenagerswithautism.com
- Son-Rise – www.autismtreatmentcenter.org
- Center for Autism Research and Development (CARD) – www.centerforautism.com
- Relationship Development Intervention (RDI) – www.rdiconnect.com

Diet Information Resources

- Autism Network for Dietary Intervention – www.AutismNDI.com
- Talk About Curing Autism – www.tacanow.org
- Nourishing Hope – www.nourishinghope.com
- Gluten Free, Casein Free Diet – www.gfcfdiet.com
- SCD Diet – www.pecanbread.com
- Gut and Psychology Syndrome Diet (GAPS) – www.gapsdiet.com
- Feingold Diet – www.feingold.org
- Ketogenic Diet – www.ketogenicdiet.org
- Body Ecology Diet – www.bodyecology.com
- Rotation Diet – www.food-allergy.org/rotation.html

Specialty Food Resources

- Cause You're Special – www.causeyourespecial.com
- Really Great Food Company – www.reallygreatfood.com
- Gluten Free Mall – www.glutenfreemall.com
- Kinnikinnick Foods – www.kinnikinnick.com
- Gluten Solutions – www.glutensolutions.com
- Gluten Free Pantry – www.glutenfreepantry.com
- Enjoy Life Foods – www.enjoylifefoods.com
- Corganic – www.corganic.com

IEP Resources

- Wright's Law – www.wrightslaw.com
- IEP for you – www.IEP4u.com
- Talk About Curing Autism – www.tacanow.org
- *The Complete IEP Guide* by Lawrence Siegel (a must have book before beginning the IEP process)
- Education and Behavior – www.educationandbehavior.com
- Educational Learning and Training – www.iephelp.com

Lab Resources*

- Immunotech – www.immunotechlab.com
- Doctors Data – www.doctorsdata.com
- Great Plains Laboratory – www.greatplainslaboratory.com
- Quest Diagnostics – www.questdiagnostics.com
- Enterolab – www.enterolab.com
- 23 and Me – www.23andme.com

* Most labs are ordered by the physician, who uses a variety of different laboratories. The ones listed here (other than 23 and Me) are those most often used in the autism biomedical community.

Nutritional Supplement Resources

- Kirkman Laboratories – www.kirkmanlabs.com
- BrainChild Nutritionals – www.brainchildnutritionals.com
- Nordic Naturals – www.nordicnaturals.com
- Twin Lab – www.twinlab.com
- Enzymedica – www.enzymedica.com
- Immunotec – www.immunotec.com
- Our Kids ASD – www.ourkidsasd.com
- Lee Silsby – www.leesilsby.com
- Houston Enzymes – www.houstonenzymes.com
- Metagenics – www.metagenics.com

Physician Resources*

- Medical Academy of Pediatric Special Needs – www.medmaps.org
- Generation Rescue – www.generationrescue.org/find-a-physician
- Talk About Curing Autism – www.tacanow.org
- My Autism Team – www.myautismteam.com
- Naturopathic physicians – www.naturopathic.org
- Functional medicine physicians – www.functionalmedicine.org

*Research providers before making an appointment, including their expertise, years of working with children with autism, and whether or not they take insurance, since many do not.

Sibling Support

- Sibling Support Project – www.siblingsupport.org
- The Child Study Center – www.aboutourkids.org/Siblings_children_special_needs
- The Arc – www.thearc.org/siblings
- Sibling Leadership Network – www.siblingleadership.org
- University of Michigan Health System – www.med.umich.edu/yourchild/topics/specneed.htm
- Sibs – www.sibs.org.uk

Sleep Support

- National Autism Resources – www.nationalautismresources.com/autism-and-sleep
- Talk About Curing Autism – www.tacanow.org/family-resources/sleep-issues-and-asd
- Autism Speaks – www.autismspeaks.org/family-services/health-and-wellness/sleep
- Synapse Australia – www.autism-help.org/behavior-sleep-autism.htm

Specific Treatments and Therapies

- Sound Therapy – www.tomatis.com, www.berardaitwebsite.com
- Sensory Integration – www.mendability.com, www.spd-foundation.net, www.brainbalancecenters.com
- Hyperbaric Oxygen – www.hbot.com
- Homeopathy Remedies – www.nationalcenterforhomeopathy.org
- Essential Oils – There are many websites for products but no one single resource for information on essential oils and autism.
- GcMAF – www.gcmaf.eu
- IVIG – There is no one resource with a focus on IVIG but there are many references to its use in treating autism in some children.
- Chelation – Refer to general information resources
- Hippotherapy – www.americanhippotherapyassociation.org
- Vision Therapy – www.visiontherapy.org
- Speech Therapy – www.asha.org
- Occupational Therapy – www.aota.org
- Physical therapy – Refer to general information resources
- Cranial Sacral Therapy – www.upledger.com
- Chiropractic – Refer to general information resources

Apps for autism therapy – There are so many apps now for autism therapy and augmentative communication that it is difficult to single out any specific one. It is best to ask your child's therapists which apps they recommend to compliment activities they are doing in session. Therapy models have changed dramatically thanks to these new technologies. Of value to research are any that are free and pertain to autism, speech models, education, social skills, and social stories.

Bibliography

Adams, Christina. *A Real Boy: A True Story of Autism, Early Intervention, and Recovery*. New York: Berkley, 2005.

Conroy, Helen, and Lisa Joyce Goes. *The Thinking Moms' Revolution: Autism beyond the Spectrum: Inspiring True Stories from Parents Fighting to Rescue Their Children*. New York: Skyhorse Pub., 2013.

Fein, Deborah, Marriane Barton, Inge-Marie Eigsti, Elizabeth Kelley, Letitia Naigles, Robert T. Schultz, Michael Stevens, Molly Helt, Alyssa Orinstein, Michael Rosenthal, Eva Troyb, and Katherine Tyson. "Optimal Outcome in Individuals with a History of Autism." *Journal of Child Psychology and Psychiatry* 54, no. 2 (2013): 195–205. DOI: 10.1111/jcpp.12037.

Gottman, John Mordechai, and Nan Silver. *The Seven Principles for Making Marriage Work*. New York: Crown, 1999.

Hinds, Marcia. *I Know You're in There: Winning Your War against Autism*. Los Angeles: Hindsight Press, 2014.

Barry Kaufman and Raun Kaufman. *Son-Rise: The Miracle Continues*. Novato, CA : HJ Kramer, 1995.

Kaufman, Raun. *Autism Breakthrough: The Groundbreaking Method That Has Helped Families All over the World*. New York: St. Martin's Press, 2014.

Kennedy Krieger Institute. "80 Percent Autism Divorce Rate Debunked in First-of-Its Kind Scientific Study." May 19, 2010. http://www.kennedykrieger.org/overview/news/80-percent-autism-divorce-rate-debunked-first-its-kind-scientific-study#footnote.

Kübler-Ross, Elisabeth. *On Death and Dying*. New York: Macmillan, 1969.

Lauer, Vaughn. *When the School Says No, How to Get the Yes!: Securing Special Education Services for Your Child*. London: Jessica Kingsley Publications, 2013

Lewis, Lisa S. *Special Diets for Special Kids: Understanding and Implementing a Gluten and Casein Free Diet to Aid in the*

Treatment of Autism and Related Developmental Disorders. Arlington, TX: Future Horizons, 1998.

Lewis, Lisa S. *Special Diets for Special Kids. New! More Great Tasting Recipes & Tips for Implementing Special Diets to Aid in the Treatment of Autism and Related Developmental Disorders.* Arlington, TX: Future Horizons Incorporated, 2001.

Maloney, Beth A. *Saving Sammy: A Mother's Fight to Cure Her Son's OCD.* New York: Broadway Books, 2010.

Maurice, Catherine. *Let Me Hear Your Voice: A Family's Triumph Over Autism.* New York: Ballantine Books, 1994.

McCandless, Jaquelyn, Teresa Binstock, and Jack Zimmerman. *Children with Starving Brains: A Medical Treatment Guide for Autism Spectrum Disorder.* Thousand Oaks, CA: Bramble, 2009.

Meyer, Donald J., and Emily Holl. *The Sibling Survival Guide: Indispensable Information for Brothers and Sisters of Adults with Disabilities.* Bethesda, MD: Woodbine House, 2014.

Meyer, Donald J. The Sibling Support Project. "What Siblings Would Like Parents and Service Providers to Know." http://www.siblingsupport.org/publications/what-siblings-would-like-parents-and-service-providers-to-know.

Seroussi, Karyn. *Unraveling the Mystery of Autism and Pervasive Developmental Disorder: A Mother's Story of Research and Recovery.* New York: Simon & Schuster, 2000.

Siri, Ken, and Tony Lyons. *Cutting-Edge Therapies for Autism, Fourth Edition.* New York: Skyhorse Pub., 2014.

Smith, Manuel J. *When I Say No, I Feel Guilty: How to Cope— using the Skills of Systematic Assertive Therapy.* New York: Dial, 1975.

Siegel, Lawrence M. *The Complete IEP Guide: How to Advocate for your Special Ed Child.* California: NOLO, 2014.

Acknowledgments

There is a reason why some of my dearest friends have come from our journey to help our children. We are each other's confidants, sources of wisdom, and the constant reminders that we are not alone. Ever.

To all of the parents, physicians, therapists, educators, and supportive strangers my family and I have met on this autism journey over the years, know that not a day goes by that I don't realize the impact you made in our lives. Specifically, I thank those professionals who were with us in the early days after the diagnosis, including Charlotte Feichtmann, Debbie Garcia, Dr. Sudhir Gupta, Diane Campbell, Nina Welch, and Monique Welch.

Thanks to all of the leaders in our community who are making a difference just by possessing the seven traits of a bold parent, and for being examples for the rest of us to follow. To my fellow TACA coordinators and to Lisa Ackerman, I owe you all more than you know. Thank you for teaching me and inspiring me to find the answers for Daniel. This book, then, is a testament to the possibilities that exist for a better future for our community.

To those who allowed me to tell your stories—Cindy, Lori, Tracey, Lisa R., Amanda, Carolyn, Julia, Sarah, Erin, Christine, Kim, Shelly, Mary Beth, Jennifer, Raun, Christina, Leah, Marcia, Terri, and the others who are mentioned anecdotally but not by name—thank you. To the fearless parents in our community who are quietly making a difference in their own families, and then reaching out to help the next family in need. You are braver than you know.

I must acknowledge Don Meyer, founder of the Sibling Support Project, Dr. Jamell White, Jonah Green, and Sarah Norris for their work with families and the siblings of children with special needs. A special shout-out to Natalie Palumbo for being the best advocate her brother Anthony could ever have.

My gratitude to Teri Arranga for her encouragement when I hesitated in submitting the proposal for the book, along with prodding the effort along the way. You are persistent, my friend.

Thank you to the staff at Skyhorse Publishing for your dedication and effort in bringing this book to fruition in record time. In particular, thank you Tony Lyons, Julia Abramoff, and my editor Andres Dietz-Chavez.

Thank you to my agent Susan Lee Cohen, who was the first to have faith in me and the message in this book, over seven years ago (hard to believe it took that long). Her grace and patience allowed me to finally bring this book to publication.

I am incredibly appreciative of my work colleagues at *The Grafton News*, who gave me back my love of writing when I needed it the most. Thank you Don, Wendy, and Cindy for the chance to report on events in town and to discover that the written word still has the power to persuade.

To my family, who experienced many nights of foraging through leftovers for dinner because Mom was too busy writing. Thank you to my husband Rich for his unwavering support of this book, to my daughter Theresa for her beauty inside and out, to Daniel for helping me find my "mission," and to David for reminding me to laugh each and every day.

My deepest gratitude and thanks to Dr. Anju Usman, MD, for writing the foreword to this book. It is an honor to have her join us in providing testimony to what our families and children endure, and the ways we intend to heal as individuals and as a community.

And finally, my love, tears, and entire sense of purpose is filled by the children affected by autism, both the children with autism and their siblings. As your parents and caregivers, we owe you so much for the ways you have shaped and changed us to be better people, because of our love for you. For the children who have died in our community due to wandering, seizures, mitochondrial disorder, immune system dysfunction, and vaccine injury, we will never forget why the battle for better health is not in vain.

Mary Romaniec, 2015

6/14/16